Prevention of Diabetes

EDITED BY

Peter Schwarz MD, PhD

Head, Division for Prevention and Care of Diabetes Mellitus
Department of Medicine III
University of Dresden
Dresden, Germany

Prasuna Reddy BA, MA, PhD, MAPS

Professor and Director CRRMH
School of Medicine and Public Health
University of Newcastle
Callaghan, NSW, Australia

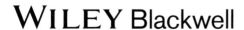

This edition first published 2013 © 2013 by John Wiley & Sons, Ltd.

Registered office: John Wiley & Sons, Ltd, The Atrium, Southern Gate, Chichester, West Sussex, PO19 8SQ, UK

Editorial offices: 9600 Garsington Road, Oxford, OX4 2DQ, UK
The Atrium, Southern Gate, Chichester, West Sussex, PO19 8SQ, UK
111 River Street, Hoboken, NJ 07030-5774, USA

For details of our global editorial offices, for customer services and for information about how to apply for permission to reuse the copyright material in this book please see our website at www. wiley.com/wiley-blackwell

Library of Congress Cataloging-in-Publication Data
Prevention of diabetes / edited by Peter Schwarz, Prasuna Reddy.
   p. ; cm.
  Includes bibliographical references and index.
  ISBN 978-0-470-65465-1 (pbk. : alk. paper) – ISBN 978-1-118-66129-1 (ePDF) – ISBN 978-1-118-66130-7 (Mobi) – ISBN 978-1-118-66131-4 (ePub) – ISBN 978-1-118-66132-1
  I. Schwarz, Peter (Physician) II. Reddy, Prasuna.
  [DNLM: 1. Diabetes Mellitus, Type 2–prevention & control. 2. Diabetes Mellitus, Type 2– complications. 3. Diabetes Mellitus, Type 2–diagnosis. 4. Evidence-Based Medicine–education. 5. Risk Factors.   WK 810]
  RC660.4
  616.4′62–dc23
                   2013013319

A catalogue record for this book is available from the British Library.

Wiley also publishes its books in a variety of electronic formats. Some content that appears in print may not be available in electronic books.

Cover image: © Garth Stewart; © Shutterstock / eltoro69; iStockPhoto / dutch icon
Cover design by Garth Stewart

Set in 9.5/13 pt Meridien by Toppan Best-set Premedia Limited
Printed and bound in Singapore by Ho Printing Singapore Pte Ltd

01   2013

Contents

Contributors

Abdul Basit MBBS, FRCP(Lon)
Director, Baqai Institute of Diabetology and
Endocrinology (BIDE)
Professor of Medicine
Baqai Medical University
Karachi, Pakistan

Michael Bergman MD, FACP
Clinical Professor of Medicine
NYU School of Medicine
Division of Endocrinology
NYU Diabetes and Endocrine Associates
New York, NY, USA

Bishwajit Bhowmik MBBS, DDM
Research Fellow – Diabetes
Institute of Health and Society
Faculty of Medicine
University of Oslo; *and*
Manager, Diabetes Prevention Intervention
Study (DPIS)
Oslo, Norway

Martin Buysschaert MD, PhD
Professor of Medicine
Head of the Department
Université Catholique de Louvain (UCL)
University Clinic Saint-Luc
Department of Endocrinology and Diabetology
Brussels, Belgium

Avivit Cahn MD
Attending Physician
Endocrinology and Metabolism Service; *and*
The Diabetes Unit
Department of Medicine
Hadassah-Hebrew University Medical Center
Jerusalem, Israel

Stephen Colagiuri MD
Professor of Metabolic Health
Boden Institute of Obesity, Nutrition, Exercise,
and Eating Disorders
University of Sydney
Sydney, NSW, Australia

Emmanuel Cosson MD, PhD
Professor
Department of Endocrinology Diabetology
Nutrition
Jean Verdier Hospital, AP-HP
Paris Nord University, CRNH-IdF
Bondy, France

Melanie Davies MD
Professor of Diabetes Medicine
Diabetes Research Unit
College of Medicine, Biological
Sciences and Psychology
University of Leicester
Leicester, UK

Martin R. Fischer MD, MME (Berne)
Professor of Internal Medicine and Medical
Education
Department of Medical Education
Munich University Hospital
Munich, Germany

Alice Gibson BSc
Research Officer
Boden Institute of Obesity, Nutrition, Exercise
and Eating Disorders
University of Sydney
Sydney, NSW, Australia

Aleksandra Gilis-Januszewska
Chair, Department of Endocrinology
Collegium Medicum, Jagiellonian University
Krakow, Poland

Norbert Hermanns PhD
Professor of Clinical Psychology
Department of Clinical Psychology, University
of Bamberg, Bamberg; *and*
Director, Research Institute of Diabetes
Academy Mergentheim (FIDAM)
Bad Mergentheim, Germany

Akhtar Hussain MD, PhD, DSc
Professor of Chronic Diseases – Diabetes
Institute of Health and Society, Faculty of
Medicine
University of Oslo; *and*
Coordinator, Diabetes Prevention Intervention
Study (DPIS)
Oslo, Norway

Baruch Itzhak MD
Specialist in Family Medicine
Israel National Diabetes Prevention Committee
Jerusalem, Israel

**Greg Johnson B Pharm, Dip Hosp
Pharm, MBA**
Chief Executive Officer
Diabetes Australia
Adjunct Professor, Faculty of Health
Deakin University
Melbourne, VIC, Australia

Kamlesh Khunti MD, PhD
Professor of Primary Care Diabetes and
Vascular Medicine
Diabetes Research Unit
College of Medicine, Biological
Sciences and Psychology
University of Leicester
Leicester, UK

Peter Kronsbein PhD
Professor of Counselling and Nutrition
Education
Niederrhein University of Applied Sciences
Faculty of Nutrition, Food, and Hospitality
Sciences
Mönchengladbach, Germany

Rüdiger Landgraf MD
Professor of Internal Medicine, Endocrinology
and Diabetology
German Diabetes Foundation
Munich, Germany

Stavros Liatis MD
Senior Consultant in Internal Medicine and
Diabetology
First Department of Propaedeutic Medicine
Athens University Medical School
Laiko General Hospital
Athens, Greece

Jaana Lindström PhD
Research Manager
Department of Chronic Disease Prevention
Diabetes Prevention Unit
National Institute for Health and Welfare (THL)
Helsinki, Finland

**Konstantinos Makrilakis MD, MPH,
PhD**
Assistant Professor of Internal Medicine
First Department of Propaedeutic Medicine
Athens University Medical School
Laiko General Hospital
Athens, Greece

**Andrew Milat BHMS Ed (Hons),
MPH (Hons)**
Associate Director, Evidence and Evaluation
New South Wales (NSW) Ministry of Health
North Sydney, NSW, Australia

Markku Peltonen PhD
Director and Adjunct Professor
Department of Chronic Disease Prevention
National Institute for Health and Welfare (THL)
Helsinki, Finland

Itamar Raz MD
Professor of Medicine
The Diabetes Unit, Department of Medicine
Hadassah-Hebrew University Medical Center
Jerusalem, Israel

Prasuna Reddy BA, MA, PhD, MAPS
Professor and Director CRRMH
School of Medicine and Public Health
University of Newcastle
Callaghan, NSW, Australia

Musarrat Riaz MBBS, FCPS
Consultant Diabetologist
Baqai Institute of Diabetology & Endocrinology
(BIDE)
Karachi, Pakistan

Peter Schwarz MD, PhD
Head, Division for Prevention and Care of
Diabetes Mellitus
Department of Medicine III
University of Dresden
Dresden, Germany

Jane Shill BSc, MSc
Evaluation and Research Coordinator
Life! program
Diabetes Australia – Victoria
Melbourne, VIC, Australia

Victoria Telle Hjellset PhD
Post Doctoral Fellow
Institute of General Practice and Community
Medicine
Department of Preventive Medicine and
Epidemiology
University of Oslo and
Norwegian University of Life Sciences
Oslo, Norway

Amy Timoshanko PhD
Prevention and Health Promotion Manager
Diabetes Australia – Victoria
Melbourne, VIC, Australia

**Daniel Tolks
Diplom-Gesundheitswirt**
Research Fellow
Department of Medical Education
Munich University Hospital
Munich, Germany

Paul Valensi MD
Professor, Head of the Department
Department of Endocrinology Diabetology
Nutrition
Jean Verdier Hospital, AP-HP
Paris Nord University, CRNH-IdF
Bondy, France

Philip Vita BSc, MAppPsych
Director, Sydney Diabetes Prevention Program
Boden Institute of Obesity, Nutrition, Exercise
and Eating Disorders
University of Sydney and Sydney Local Health
District
Sydney, NSW, Australia

Thomas Yates PhD
Senior Lecturer in Physical Activity
Sedentary Behaviour and Health Diabetes
Research Unit
College of Medicine, Biological
Sciences and Psychology
University of Leicester
Leicester, UK

Preface

Noncommunicable diseases represent a great and growing threat to health and development worldwide. Four of these diseases: cancers, diabetes, cardiovascular diseases, and chronic respiratory diseases, are currently responsible for 60% of all deaths globally, with 80% in low and middle-income countries.

Diabetes is particularly challenging as it is increasing rapidly. The International Diabetes Federation predicts that in the next 17 years, the number of people worldwide living with diabetes will increase from 285 million to 552 million. Diabetes is a disease of poverty; it is increasing most rapidly in poor vulnerable populations and resource-poor settings. A large segment of the world's population is at high risk of diabetes, but only a very small proportion are screened or diagnosed.

Yet diabetes, like cardiovascular diseases and cancers, is largely preventable. Up to 80% of heart disease, stroke, and type 2 diabetes could be prevented by eliminating shared risk factors, mainly tobacco use, unhealthy diet, and physical inactivity. While sedentary behavior and poor nutrition, especially excessive consumption of calories, salt, saturated fat and sugar, increase the risk of noncommunicable diseases, there is good evidence that healthful diets and regular physical activity can reduce the risk of diabetes and cardiovascular disease.

The chapters in this book are examples of translational research, intervention trials, practical programs and designs required to address key challenges in the global action to prevent diabetes.

The identification of target populations for intervention is the theme of a chapter from Paris Nord University researchers. They describe a screening strategy for identifying glycemic abnormalities to detect prediabetes and type 2 diabetes. Researchers Buysschaert and Bergman from Belgium and the US respectively, discuss diagnosis of prediabetes and diabetes prevention. They focus on the status of diagnostic criteria related to glucose and more recently HbA1c levels. The development of quality and outcome standards for diabetes prevention is the topic of a chapter by Peltonen and Landgraf. They provide important information on quality indicators and outcome evaluation indicators that allow for measurement and comparative evaluation of different diabetes prevention approaches.

The comorbidity of diabetes and depression is the topic of a chapter by Hermanns. This renowned researcher discusses the advantages of a structured diabetes prevention program that also addresses psychological aspects of lifestyle modification. The role of physical activity in prevention of type 2 diabetes is covered in a chapter by researchers from the University of Leicester. The authors describe ways of initiating physical activity behavior change and the implications of the sedentary behavior paradigm.

A community-based lifestyle prevention program for prevention of diabetes is described in a chapter by a team of researchers from Greece, Poland, and Germany. The evaluation of the program in cohorts in two different communities and countries, showed improvement in cardiovascular risk factors and benefits in weight loss. A team of researchers from Israel has provided a chapter describing implementation of diabetes prevention programs directed at two levels: high risk populations and whole populations. The chapter emphasizes creating health promoting environments and quality improvement of interventional programs.

Implementing diabetes prevention programs in South Asia raises a particular set of challenges that are discussed by researchers from Pakistan. They describe the need for multidisciplinary teams to be active in primary prevention, and public health campaigns focused on children and adolescents. Another chapter considers the epidemiologic trends of diabetes among Asian Indians and migrant South Asians. The authors note that government prevention policy needs to consider training of healthcare practitioners in effective strategies for migrant groups.

An Australian team has looked closely at recruitment and retention in diabetes prevention programs. They describe the difficulties and possible solutions of attracting high risk participants into government-funded group programs, and note the under-representation of men and the socially disadvantaged. Training health professionals in diabetes prevention using new media is discussed by Tolles and Fischer from Germany. They provide an intriguing overview of e-learning approaches, web technologies, and the uses of new media in health promotion and diabetes prevention.

The chapters in this book represent advances in the application of research to address the prevention of diabetes, and more broadly, the prevention of noncommunicable diseases, which account for a large share of the global disease burden.

Professor Peter Schwarz
Professor Prasuna Reddy

CHAPTER 1

What have we learned from the number of clinical trials?

Jaana Lindström

Department of Chronic Disease Prevention, Diabetes Prevention Unit, National Institute for Health and Welfare (THL), Helsinki, Finland

Introduction

The primary prevention of type 2 diabetes (T2D) was originally proposed by Dr. E. Joslin in 1921 [1]. He commented on how obese people are more likely to have diabetes than their slimmer neighbors. Indeed, to be able to prevent a chronic disease such as T2D it is necessary to have knowledge about its modifiable risk factors and natural history. Furthermore, there should be a preclinical phase or a "window of opportunity" for intervention as well as a feasible screening tool to identify high-risk individuals. In addition, the efficacy of the intervention has to be proven in a clinical trial setting.

T2D is a very expensive disease – about 10–15% of the total health care costs in developed countries are spent to treat T2D and, in particular, its complications [2,3]. To avoid late complications of T2D and related costs, prevention of T2D itself is therefore desirable. There are some "natural" experiments in which ethnic groups have experienced rapid westernization and with it a rapid increase in the rates of obesity and T2D [4]. Therefore it is logical to assume that by reversing these lifestyle changes it would be possible to prevent the development of the disease. Such a potential for reversibility has been shown among Australian Aboriginals [5]. In these experiments hyperglycemic people returned to living in a traditional hunter–gatherer way of life – an ultimate lifestyle change not suitable for everybody.

T2D develops as a result of complex multifactorial process with both lifestyle and genetic origins. The main risk factors for T2D are obesity and

Prevention of Diabetes, First Edition. Edited by Peter Schwarz and Prasuna Reddy.
© 2013 John Wiley & Sons, Ltd. Published 2013 by John Wiley & Sons, Ltd.

a sedentary lifestyle [6]. A "westernized" dietary pattern with low fiber [7–9] and high saturated [10] and trans fats [11], refined carbohydrates [12], sweetened beverages [13], sodium [14], and red meat and processed meat products [15,16] intake has been shown to be associated with increased T2D risk. Another feature of modern lifestyle, voluntary sleep deprivation, also increases diabetes risk [17,18]. Protective lifestyle factors, in addition to those mentioned above, include coffee [19–21] and moderate alcohol, particularly wine consumption [22].

Impaired glucose tolerance (IGT) is a hyperglycemic state between normoglycemia and T2D, diagnosed by a 2-h oral glucose tolerance test (OGTT). Of the people with IGT, approximately half will develop T2D during a 10-year follow-up period [23,24]. In Asian populations the rate of progression seems to be even faster [25,26]. It is well known that the risk of complications begins in the prediabetic phase prior to glucose levels reaching diagnostic cut-points for T2D [27–29]. People with IGT would thus be the perfect subjects for preventive interventions.

Major lifestyle trials in prevention of T2D

Da-Qing Study
A large population-based screening program (110 660 persons screened with OGTT) to identify people with IGT was carried out in Da-Qing, China, in 1986 [25,30]. The randomization of study subjects was not random, but the 33 participating clinics (= cluster randomization) were randomized to carry out the intervention according to one of the four specified intervention protocols (diet alone, exercise alone, diet–exercise combined, or none). Altogether, 577 (312 men, 264 women + 1 undefined) subjects with IGT participated in the trial, and of these 533 participated in the measurements at the end of the intervention in 1992. The cumulative 6-year incidence of T2D was lower in the three intervention groups (diet alone, exercise alone, diet–exercise combined; 41–46%) than the control group (68%). Because no individual allocation of study subjects to the intervention and control groups was done, the results based on individual data analysis must be interpreted with caution. The study subjects were relatively lean, with a mean body mass index (BMI) of 25.8 kg/m^2, but, despite that, the progression from IGT to diabetes was high; more than 10% per year in the control group.

In clinics assigned to dietary intervention, the participants were encouraged to reduce weight if their BMI was >25 kg/m^2, aiming at <24 kg/m^2, otherwise a high carbohydrate (55–65 energy proportion (E%)) and moderate fat (25–30E%) diet was recommended. Participants were encouraged to consume more vegetables, reduce simple sugar intake, and control alcohol intake. Small group counseling sessions concerning diet and/or physical activity were organized weekly for the first month, monthly for 3 months, and every 3 months thereafter. Participants also received individual counseling by physicians. The participants were encouraged to increase their level of leisure time physical activity by at least 1–2 "units" per day, one unit corresponding to 30 minutes of slow walking, shopping, house cleaning, or traveling by bus, 20 minutes of cycling or ballroom dancing, 10 minutes of slow running, climbing stairs, or disco dancing, or 5 minutes of swimming, jumping rope, or playing basketball.

The overall changes in risk factor patterns were relatively small. Body weight did not change in lean subjects, and there was a modest, <1 kg, reduction in subjects with baseline BMI >25 kg/m^2. The estimated changes in habitual dietary nutrient intakes were small and nonsignificant between groups. Within the exercise and diet plus exercise groups, physical activity increased modestly but statistically significantly (+ 0.6–0.8 activity units per day on average). Thus, it is not easy to determine the factors responsible for the beneficial effects on the risk of T2D. In this population, weight control obviously was not the key issue. Physical activity and qualitative changes in diet that are difficult to measure on individual level probably played a key part.

The 20-year follow-up of the original study cohort [30] showed that the reduction in diabetes incidence persisted in the combined intervention group compared with control participants with no intervention, and, furthermore, the risk reduction remained essentially the same during the post-intervention period. It should be noted that diabetes incidence during the follow-up was high: in the final analyses 80% of the intervention participants and 93% of the control participants had developed diabetes. The follow-up analyses showed no statistically significant differences in cardiovascular disease (CVD) events, CVD mortality, or total mortality between the control group and the combined intervention groups. A non-significant 17% reduction in CVD death was observed, which can be seen to be at least suggestively in favor of the lifestyle intervention.

Finnish Diabetes Prevention Study

The intervention of the Finnish Diabetes Prevention Study (DPS) was carried out during 1993–2001 in five clinics in Finland, aiming to prevent T2D with lifestyle modification alone [24,31–33]. A total of 522 individuals at high risk of developing diabetes were recruited into the study, mainly by screening for IGT in middle-aged (age 40–64 years) overweight (BMI >25 kg/m^2) subjects. The presence of IGT before randomization was confirmed in two successive 75-g OGTT; the mean of the two values had to be within the IGT range to qualify for the study. The participants were randomly allocated either into the control group or the intensive intervention group. The subjects in the intervention group had frequent consultation visits with a nutritionist (seven times during the first year and every 3 months thereafter). They received individual advice about how to achieve the intervention goals which were reduction in weight of 5% or more, total fat intake <30% of energy consumed, saturated fat intake <10% of energy consumed, fiber intake of at least 15 g/1000 kcal, and moderate exercise for 30 minutes per day or more. Frequent consumption of wholegrain cereal products, vegetables, berries and fruit, low-fat milk and meat products, soft margarines, and vegetable oils rich in monounsaturated fatty acids were recommended. The dietary advice was based on 3-day food records completed four times per year. The participants were also individually guided to increase their level of physical activity. Endurance exercise (walking, jogging, swimming, aerobic ball games, skiing) was recommended to increase aerobic capacity and cardiorespiratory fitness. Supervised, progressive, individually tailored circuit-type resistance training sessions to improve the functional capacity and strength of the large muscle groups were also offered.

The control group participants were given only general advice about healthy lifestyle at baseline. An OGTT was carried out annually for all participants and if either fasting or 2-h glucose values reached diabetic levels a confirmatory OGTT was performed. The study end-point was only recorded if the second test also reached diabetic levels; otherwise the subjects continued with their randomized treatment.

Body weight reduction from baseline was on average 4.5 kg in the intervention group and 1.0 kg in the control group subjects ($P<0.001$) after the first year and at 3 years, weight reductions were 3.5 and 0.9 kg ($P < 0.001$), respectively. Indicators of central adiposity and glucose tolerance improved significantly more in the intervention group than in the control group at both 1-year and 3-year follow-up examinations. At the 1-year and 3-year examinations intervention group subjects reported significantly more beneficial changes in their dietary and exercise habits, based on dietary and exercise diaries.

After 4 years the cumulative incidence of diabetes was 11% (95% CI 6–15%) in the intervention group and 23% (95% CI 17–29%) in the control group. Based on life-table analysis, the risk of diabetes was reduced by 58% ($P < 0.001$) during the trial in the intervention group compared with the control group during a mean follow-up time of 3.2 years. The absolute risk reduction was 12% at that point and the number needed to treat (NNT) was 8. Both men and women benefited from lifestyle intervention: the incidence of diabetes was reduced by 63% and in women by 54% in the intervention group compared with the control group. None of the people (either in the intervention or control group) who had succeeded in achieving all five predefined lifestyle targets developed diabetes, while approximately one-third of the people who did not reach a single one of the targets developed T2D. This is direct empirical proof that the reduction of the diabetes risk was indeed mediated through the lifestyle changes. *Post hoc* analyses have also shown that both dietary changes – adopting a diet with moderate fat and high fiber content [34] – as well as increasing physical activity [35] were independently associated with diabetes risk reduction. Furthermore, a subgroup analysis with intravenous glucose tolerance testing (n = 87 at baseline and 52 at 4-year examination) showed improvement in insulin resistance which was highly correlated with achieved body weight reduction [36]. The effect of lifestyle intervention on diabetes incidence was shown to be the largest among the oldest age group and those with the highest baseline risk profile, as measured with the Finnish Diabetes Risk Score (FINDRISC) [37].

An analysis using the data collected during the extended follow-up of the DPS revealed that after a median of 7 years' total follow-up a marked reduction in the cumulative incidence of diabetes was sustained [24]. The relative risk reduction during the total follow-up was 43%. The effect of intervention on diabetes risk was maintained among those who after the intervention period were without diabetes: after median post-intervention follow-up time of 3 years the corresponding incidence rates were 4.6 and 7.2 per 100 person-years, respectively (log-rank test $P = 0.0401$), that is, 36% relative risk reduction.

The 10-year follow-up results on the effect of DPS lifestyle intervention on total mortality and cardiovascular morbidity were published in 2009 [38], based on register linkage of the original study cohort to the national Hospital Discharge Register and Death Register. Among the DPS participants who consented for register linkage (n = 505), total mortality (2.2 vs. 3.8 per 1000 person-years) and cardiovascular morbidity (22.9 vs. 22.0 per 1000 person-years) were similar in the intervention and control groups. Interestingly, when the DPS intervention and control groups together were compared with a population-based cohort including people with IGT, adjusted hazard ratios were 0.21 (95% CI 0.09–0.52) and 0.39 (95% CI 0.20–0.79) for total mortality and 0.89 (95% CI 0.62–1.27) and 0.87 (95% CI 0.60–1.27) for cardiovascular morbidity. Thus, the risk of death among the DPS participants was markedly lower than in a population-based IGT cohort.

Diabetes Prevention Program

The Diabetes Prevention Program (DPP) [39,40] was a multicenter randomized clinical trial carried out in the United States. It compared the efficacy and safety of three interventions: an intensive lifestyle intervention or standard lifestyle recommendations combined with metformin or placebo. The study focused on high-risk individuals (n = 3234) with IGT who also had slightly elevated fasting plasma glucose (>5.5 mmol/L). The main results were intensive lifestyle intervention reduced T2D risk after 2.8 years' mean follow-up by 58% compared with the placebo control group. Lifestyle intervention was also shown to be superior to metformin treatment (850 mg twice daily) which led to T2D risk reduction of 31% compared with placebo [39].

The lifestyle intervention in DPP was primarily carried out by special educators, "case managers" and was relatively intense. The lifestyle intervention commenced with a 16-session structured core curriculum within the first 24 weeks after randomization, followed by individual sessions with the case manager every 2 months. The goals of the dietary intervention were to achieve and maintain a 7% weight reduction by consuming a healthy, low-calorie, low-fat diet and to engage in physical activities of moderate intensity (such as brisk walking) 150 minutes per week or more. Clinical centers (n = 27) also offered supervised activity sessions where attendance was voluntary. Of the DPP participants assigned to intensive lifestyle intervention, 74% achieved the study goal of ≥150 minutes of activity per week at 24 weeks. At 1-year visit the mean weight loss was 7 kg (about 7%).

The DPP investigators have also attempted to clarify the relative contributions of different components of the lifestyle intervention to the reduction in diabetes incidence in the intensive lifestyle intervention arm of the DPP [41]. Furthermore, they aimed to assess the contribution of diet and activity changes on weight loss. The main finding was that body weight at baseline and weight reduction during the intervention were the most important predictors of diabetes risk. Lower weight (10 kg) at baseline resulted in a 12% lower diabetes incidence, even when adjusted for demographics and changes in dietary fat intake and physical activity. For each kilogram lost, the risk of developing diabetes was estimated to be reduced by 16%. In the model assessing one intervention characteristic at a time, the energy proportion of fat was a significant predictor of the incidence of diabetes, with a 5% reduction leading to a hazard ratio of 0.75 (0.63–0.88). However, in the multivariate models with predictors as continuous variables and with baseline body weight and weight reduction as covariates, neither physical activity nor energy proportion of dietary fat predicted diabetes. Nevertheless, among the participants not meeting the weight loss goal during the first year of the trial, those who achieved the physical activity goal had a 44% lower incidence of diabetes.

Indian Diabetes Prevention Program

The Indian Diabetes Prevention Program (IDPP) recruited 531 subjects with IGT (mean age 46 years, BMI 25.8 kg/m^2) who were randomized into four groups (control, lifestyle modification, metformin, and combined lifestyle modification and metformin) [26,42]. Lifestyle modification included advice on physical activity (30 minutes of brisk walking per day) and reduction in total calories, refined carbohydrates and fats, avoidance of sugar, and inclusion of fiber-rich foods. The intervention included personal sessions at baseline and 6-monthly, and monthly telephone contacts. The intensity of the intervention thus was lower than in the DPP and DPS. After a median follow-up of 30 months, the relative risk reduction was 28.5% with lifestyle modification, 26.4% with metformin, and 28.2% with lifestyle modification and metformin, compared with the control group [26]. Thus, there was no added benefit from combining the drug and lifestyle interventions. In the control group, diabetes incidence was high (55% in 3 years) and comparable to the findings from the Chinese study [25].

Japanese Prevention Trial

The Japanese Prevention Trial included 458 men who were diagnosed with IGT in health screening and allocated randomly to receive either intensive lifestyle intervention (n = 102) or standard intervention (n = 356) [43]. The participants in the intensive intervention group visited hospital every 3–4 months where they were given detailed, repeated advice to reduce body weight if their BMI was ≥22 kg/m^2 (otherwise, to maintain their weight) by consuming large amount of vegetables and reducing the total amount of other food by 10%, for example, by using a smaller rice bowl. Intake of fat (<50 g per day) and alcohol (<50 g per day) were limited, as was eating out (no more than once a day). Physical activity was recommended (30–40 min per day of walking, etc.). The participants in the control group visited hospital every 6 months and were given standard advice to eat smaller meals and increase their physical activity.

The cumulative 4-year incidence of diabetes was 3% in the intervention group and 9.3% in the control group, with 67.4% risk reduction ($P < 0.001$). BMI at baseline was 23.8 ± 2.1 in the intervention group and 24.0 ± 2.3 in the control group. Body weight decreased by 2.18 kg in the intervention group and 0.39 kg in the control group during the 4 years follow-up ($P < 0.001$). Thus, there was a remarkable reduction in diabetes risk despite the relatively modest weight reduction. *Post hoc* analyses in the control group revealed that diabetes incidence was positively correlated with change in body weight in this population; however, weight loss was not the sole explanator of diabetes risk reduction.

Other trials

Several more recent and/or smaller prevention trials have been completed, with very similar findings to the trials already presented. The SLIM Study [44,45] in the Netherlands aimed to determine the effect of diet and exercise intervention on glucose tolerance, insulin resistance, and CVD risk factors in individuals with IGT. At 3 years'follow-up among those who completed the trial (n = 106) the cumulative incidence of T2DM was 18% in the intervention group and 38% in the control group, with relative risk 0.42 ($P = 0.025$); a 58% risk reduction.

The European Diabetes Prevention Study (EDIPS) extended the DPS to other European populations, using the same study design. In the Newcastle arm of this study (EDIPS–Newcastle) [46], among 102 participants with IGT (42 men and 60 women, mean age 57 years, mean BMI 34 kg/m^2) the overall incidence of diabetes was reduced by 55% in the intervention group compared with the control group, with RR 0.45 (95% CI 0.2–1.2). These results contribute to the evidence that T2D can be prevented by lifestyle changes in adults with IGT.

The PREDIMED-Reus [47] was a substudy to a large nutrition intervention trial (the PREDIMED study) for primary cardiovascular disease prevention in persons at high risk. Altogether, 418 nondiabetic subjects aged 55–80 years were randomized to education on a low-fat diet (control group) or one of two Mediterranean diets, supplemented with either free virgin olive oil (1 L per week) or nuts (30 g per day). No advice on physical activity was given. After a median follow-up of 4.0 years, multivariable-adjusted hazard ratios of diabetes were 0.49 (0.25–0.97) and 0.48 (0.24–

0.96) in the Mediterranean diet groups supplemented with olive oil and nuts, respectively, compared with the control group. Diabetes risk reduction occurred in the absence of significant changes in body weight or physical activity.

Clinical trial evidence of the effect of lifestyle components on T2D risk

The results from clinical trials to prevent T2D have been surprisingly similar: a significant reduction in diabetes incidence has been observed following lifestyle modification. The intervention methods used to modify lifestyle have varied between the studies, because it is obvious that socio-cultural issues and the available facilities and personnel have dictated the application of the intervention. However, they have also several features in common. Lifestyle intervention in these clinical trials had a strong focus on increased physical activity (2.5–4 hours per week) and dietary modification (increased whole grain, fiber, vegetables, and fruit, reduced total and saturated fat, sugar and refined grain). Weight reduction among overweight participants was also an important goal and predictor of decreased diabetes risk in many of the studies [41]; however, beneficial changes in diabetes incidence were also achieved independently of weight reduction [25,26,47]. The interventions utilized behavior modification techniques such as motivational interviewing, self-monitoring, and individualized short and long-term goals.

In most of the published prevention trials the main aim was to explore the effect of comprehensive lifestyle intervention. In the Chinese prevention study [25] an attempt to determine whether a diet or exercise intervention is more effective revealed no difference in outcome between the two interventions.

In the DPS the risk of being diagnosed with diabetes was strongly associated with the number of lifestyle goals achieved [24]. Success in achieving the intervention goals in the DPS was estimated from the food records and exercise questionnaires. The success score (0–5) was calculated as the sum of achieved lifestyle goals. There was a strong inverse correlation between the success score and the incidence of diabetes during the total follow-up. This was especially apparent when the success in achieving the goals was assessed at year 3, which probably reflects the importance of sustained lifestyle changes. The independent effects of achieving the success score components at 3-year examination was assessed by including each of the five lifestyle goal variables individually in a Cox model. Univariate hazard ratios for diabetes incidence (95% CI) were 0.45 (0.31–0.64) for weight reduction from baseline, 0.65 (0.45–0.95) for intake of fat, 0.59 (0.31–1.13) for intake of saturated fat, 0.69 (0.49–0.96) for intake of fiber, and 0.62 (0.46–0.84) for physical activity, comparing those who did or did not achieve the respective goal. When all the five success score components were simultaneously included in the Cox model, the multivariate adjusted hazard ratios for diabetes (95% CI) were 0.43 (0.30–0.61) for weight reduction, 0.80 (0.48–1.34) for intake of fat, 0.55 (0.26–1.16) for intake of saturated fat, 0.97 (0.63–1.51) for intake of fiber, and 0.80 (0.57–1.12) for physical activity. Furthermore, weight change was significantly associated with the achievement of each of the other four lifestyle goals, and consequently, success score was strongly and inversely correlated with weight reduction [24].

Correspondingly, the reduction in body weight was reported to be the main determinant of risk reduction in the US DPP [41]. After adjusment for other components of the intervention, there was a 16% reduction in diabetes risk per 1 kg weight lost during the first year of the intervention. Furthermore, lower percentage of calories from fat and increased physical activity predicted weight loss, and increased physical activity was important to help sustain weight loss. Achieving the physical activity goal of 150 min per week reduced diabetes risk especially among those participants who did not achieve the weight reduction goal.

The findings suggest that dietary composition and physical activity are important in diabetes prevention and their effect on diabetes risk is partly but not entirely mediated through resulting weight reduction. Due to multicollinearity, the results should be interpreted cautiously. In the Indian IDPP [26] and Chinese prevention study [25] the participants were relatively lean and there was no large change in body weight, but despite that a remarkable reduction in diabetes risk was apparent. Thus, in these studies other components of the intervention than weight control were responsible for the beneficial effects on diabetes risk. In the PREDIMED-Reus study diabetes risk reduction was associated with compliance with the Mediterranean diet [47] and especially with high intake of either nuts or extra virgin olive oil. So far there have been no studies comparing the "healthy diet" based on the DPS and DPP approach (reduced saturated fat, moderate total fat, increased fiber from cereal and vegetables) with the Mediterraned diet scheme of the PREDIMED-Reus. Possibly the best solution would be a combination of both: emphasis on quality of diet but simultaneous aim of moderate weight reduction.

A pragmatic way to prevent diabetes therefore would be to focus strongly on behavioral factors such as diet composition and physical activity. Dietary changes according to the intervention goals will reduce the energy density of the diet and lead to decreased total energy intake. Increased physical activity on the other hand will increase energy consumption. Together, these changes, even if relatively modest, can lead to weight reduction. A strict diet emphasizing dietary restriction and aiming solely at weight reduction may be more efficient for achieving weight loss in the short term, but typically does not lead to sustained behavioral change.

Diets may vary according to food culture, food availability, and personal preferences, and yet follow the same general principles, as shown by the clinical studies. Based on the range of different diets associated with diabetes prevention these principles are as follow [48]:

- Aim for a high intake of vegetables
- Consume mainly unrefined, wholegrain cereal products
- Choose vegetable oils such as olive or rapeseed oil for everyday use
- Opt for fish, dairy, or vegetable sources of proteins (e.g., nuts, legumes)
- Limit the intake of highly processed or energy-dense foods that are high in fat and/or refined sugar (e.g., processed meat, sweetened beverages, confectionery).

References

1. Joslin E. The prevention of diabetes mellitus. JAMA 1921;76:79–84.
2. Haffner SM, Stern MP, Hazuda HP, Mitchell BD, Patterson JK. Cardiovascular risk factors in confirmed prediabetic individuals: does the clock for coronary heart disease start ticking before the onset of clinical diabetes? JAMA 1990;263:2893–8.
3. Harris M, Klein R, Welborn T, Knuiman M. Onset of NIDDM occurs at least 4–7 years before clinical diagnosis. Diabetes Care 1992;15:815–9.
4. Zimmet P, Alberti KG, Shaw J. Global and societal implications of the diabetes epidemic. Nature 2001;414(6865):782–7.
5. O'Dea K. Marked improvement in carbohydrate and lipid metabolism in diabetic Australian Aborigines after temporary reversion to traditional lifestyle. Diabetes 1980;33:596–603.
6. WHO Study Group. Diabetes mellitus. Technical Report Series No 727. Geneva; 1985. Report No. 727.
7. Salmeron J, Manson JE, Stampfer MJ, Colditz GA, Wing AL, Willett WC. Dietary fiber, glycemic load, and risk of non-insulin-dependent diabetes mellitus in women. JAMA 1997;277(6):472–7.
8. Schulze MB, Liu S, Rimm EB, Manson JE, Willett WC, Hu FB. Glycemic index, glycemic load, and dietary fiber intake and incidence of type 2 diabetes in younger and middle-aged women. Am J Clin Nutr 2004;80(2):348–56.

9. Montonen J, Knekt P, Järvinen R, Aromaa A, Reunanen A. Whole-grain and fiber intake and the incidence of type 2 diabetes. Am J Clin Nutr 2003;77(3):622–9.

10. Feskens EJ, Virtanen SM, Räsänen L, Tuomilehto J, Stengård J, Pekkanen J, et al. Dietary factors determining diabetes and impaired glucose tolerance: a 20-year follow-up of the Finnish and Dutch cohorts of the Seven Countries Study. Diabetes Care 1995;18(8):1104–12.

11. Salmeron J, Hu FB, Manson JE, Stampfer MJ, Colditz GA, Rimm EB, et al. Dietary fat intake and risk of type 2 diabetes in women. Am J Clin Nutr 2001;73(6):1019–26.

12. Hodge AM, English DR, O'Dea K, Giles GG. Glycemic index and dietary fiber and the risk of type 2 diabetes. Diabetes Care 2004;27(11):2701–6.

13. Schulze MB, Manson JE, Ludwig DS, Colditz GA, Stampfer MJ, Willett WC, et al. Sugar-sweetened beverages, weight gain, and incidence of type 2 diabetes in young and middle-aged women. JAMA 2004;292(8):927–34.

14. Hu G, Jousilahti P, Peltonen M, Lindstrom J, Tuomilehto J. Urinary sodium and potassium excretion and the risk of type 2 diabetes: a prospective study in Finland. Diabetologia 2005;48(8):1477–83.

15. Fung TT, Schulze M, Manson JE, Willett WC, Hu FB. Dietary patterns, meat intake, and the risk of type 2 diabetes in women. Arch Intern Med 2004;164(20):2235–40.

16. Song Y, Manson JE, Buring JE, Liu S. A prospective study of red meat consumption and type 2 diabetes in middle-aged and elderly women: the women's health study. Diabetes Care 2004;27(9):2108–15.

17. Ayas NT, White DP, Al-Delaimy WK, Manson JE, Stampfer MJ, Speizer FE, et al. A prospective study of self-reported sleep duration and incident diabetes in women. Diabetes Care 2003;26(2):380–4.

18. Mallon L, Broman J-E, Hetta J. High incidence of diabetes in men with sleep complaints or short sleep duration: a 12-year follow-up study of a middle-aged population. Diabetes Care 2005;28(11):2762–7.

19. Salazar-Martinez E, Willett WC, Ascherio A, Manson JE, Leitzmann MF, Stampfer MJ, et al. Coffee consumption and risk for type 2 diabetes mellitus. Ann Intern Med 2004;140(1):1–8.

20. Tuomilehto J, Hu G, Bidel S, Lindström J, Jousilahti P. Coffee consumption and risk of type 2 diabetes mellitus among middle-aged Finnish men and women. JAMA 2004;291(10):1213–9.

21. van Dam RM, Willett WC, Manson JE, Hu FB. Coffee, caffeine, and risk of type 2 diabetes: a prospective cohort study in younger and middle-aged US women. Diabetes Care 2006;29(2):398–403.

22. Hodge AM, English DR, O'Dea K, Giles GG. Alcohol intake, consumption pattern and beverage type, and the risk of type 2 diabetes. Diabet Med 2006;23(6):690–7.

23. Knowler WC, Narayan KM, Hanson RL, Nelson RG, Bennett PH, Tuomilehto J, et al. Preventing non-insulin-dependent diabetes. Diabetes 1995;44(5):483–8.

24. Lindström J, Ilanne-Parikka P, Peltonen M, Aunola S, Eriksson JG, Hemiö K, et al. Sustained reduction in the incidence of type 2 diabetes by lifestyle intervention: the follow-up results of the Finnish Diabetes Prevention Study. Lancet 2006;368: 1673–9.

25. Pan XR, Li GW, Hu YH, Wang JX, Yang WY, An ZX, et al. Effects of diet and exercise in preventing NIDDM in people with impaired glucose tolerance: the Da Qing IGT and Diabetes Study. Diabetes Care 1997;20:537–44.

26. Ramachandran A, Snehalatha C, Mary S, Mukesh B, Bhaskar AD, Vijay V. The Indian Diabetes Prevention Programme shows that lifestyle modification and metformin prevent type 2 diabetes in Asian Indian subjects with impaired glucose tolerance (IDPP-1). Diabetologia 2006;49(2):289–97.

27. Haffner SM, Stern MP, Hazuda HP, Mitchell BD, Patterson JK. Cardiovascular risk factors in confirmed prediabetic individuals: does the clock for coronary heart disease start ticking before the onset of clinical diabetes? JAMA 1990;263(21): 2893–8.

28. The DECODE Study Group. Glucose tolerance and cardiovascular mortality: comparison of fasting and 2-hour diagnostic criteria. Arch Intern Med 2001;161(3): 397–405.

29. Qiao Q, Jousilahti P, Eriksson J, Tuomilehto J. Predictive properties of impaired glucose tolerance for cardiovascular risk are not explained by the development of overt diabetes during follow-up. Diabetes Care 2003;26(10):2910–4.

30. Li G, Zhang P, Wang J, Gregg EW, Yang W, Gong Q, et al. The long-term effect of lifestyle interventions to prevent diabetes in the China Da Qing Diabetes Prevention Study: a 20-year follow-up study. Lancet 2008;371(9626):1783–9.

31. Tuomilehto J, Lindström J, Eriksson JG, Valle TT, Hämäläinen H, Ilanne-Parikka P, et al. Prevention of type 2 diabetes mellitus by changes in lifestyle among subjects with impaired glucose tolerance. N Engl J Med 2001;344(18):1343–50.

32. Lindström J, Louheranta A, Mannelin M, Rastas M, Salminen V, Eriksson J, et al. The Finnish Diabetes Prevention Study (DPS): lifestyle intervention and 3-year results on diet and physical activity. Diabetes Care 2003;26(12):3230–6.

33. Ilanne-Parikka P, Eriksson JG, Lindström J, Peltonen M, Aunola S, Hämäläinen H, et al. Effect of lifestyle intervention on the occurrence of metabolic syndrome and its components in the Finnish Diabetes Prevention Study. Diabetes Care 2008;31 (4):805–7.

34. Lindström J, Peltonen M, Eriksson JG, Louheranta A, Fogelholm M, Uusitupa M, et al. High-fibre, low-fat diet predicts long-term weight loss and decreased type 2 diabetes risk: the Finnish Diabetes Prevention Study. Diabetologia 2006;49(5):912–20.

35. Laaksonen DE, Lindström J, Lakka TA, Eriksson JG, Niskanen L, Wikström K, et al. Physical activity in the prevention of type 2 diabetes: the Finnish Diabetes Prevention Study. Diabetes 2005;54(1):158–65.

36. Uusitupa M, Lindi V, Louheranta A, Salopuro T, Lindstrom J, Tuomilehto J. Longterm improvement in insulin sensitivity by changing lifestyles of people with impaired glucose tolerance: 4-year results from the Finnish Diabetes Prevention Study. Diabetes 2003;52(10):2532–8.

37. Lindström J, Peltonen M, Eriksson J, Aunola S, Hämäläinen H, Ilanne-Parikka P, et al. Determinants for the effectiveness of lifestyle intervention in the Finnish Diabetes Prevention Study. Diabetes Care 2008;31(5):857–62.

38. Uusitupa M, Peltonen M, Lindström J, Aunola S, Ilanne-Parikka P, Keinänen-Kiukaanniemi S, et al. Ten-year mortality and cardiovascular morbidity in the Finnish Diabetes Prevention Study: secondary analysis of the randomized trial. PLoS ONE 2009;4(5):e5656.

39. Diabetes Prevention Program Research Group. Reduction in the incidence of type 2 diabetes with lifestyle intervention or metformin. N Engl J Med 2002;346(6): 393–403.

40. Orchard TJ, Temprosa M, Goldberg R, Haffner S, Ratner R, Marcovina S, et al. The effect of metformin and intensive lifestyle intervention on the metabolic syndrome: the Diabetes Prevention Program Randomized Trial. Ann Intern Med 2005; 142(8):611–9.

41. Hamman RF, Wing RR, Edelstein SL, Lachin JM, Bray GA, Delahanty L, et al. Effect of weight loss with lifestyle intervention on risk of diabetes. Diabetes Care 2006; 29(9):2102–7.

42. Ramachandran A, Snehalatha C, Satyavani K, Sivasankari S, Vijay V. Metabolic syndrome does not increase the risk of conversion of impaired glucose tolerance to diabetes in Asian Indians: result of Indian diabetes prevention programme. Diabetes Res Clin Pract 2007;76(2):215–8.

43. Kosaka K, Noda M, Kuzuya T. Prevention of type 2 diabetes by lifestyle intervention: a Japanese trial in IGT males. Diabetes Res Clin Pract 2005;67(2):152–62.

44. Mensink M, Feskens EJ, Saris WH, De Bruin TW, Blaak EE. Study on lifestyle intervention and impaired glucose tolerance Maastricht (SLIM): preliminary results after one year. Int J Obes Relat Metab Disord 2003;27(3):377–84.

45. Roumen C, Corpeleijn E, Feskens EJM, Mensink M, Saris WHM, Blaak EE. Impact of 3-year lifestyle intervention on postprandial glucose metabolism: the SLIM study. Diabet Med 2008;25(5):597–605.

46. Penn L, White M, Oldroyd J, Walker M, Alberti KG, Mathers JC. Prevention of type 2 diabetes in adults with impaired glucose tolerance: the European Diabetes Prevention RCT in Newcastle upon Tyne, UK. BMC Public Health 2009;9:342.

47. Salas-Salvado J, Bullo M, Babio N, Martinez-Gonzalez MA, Ibarrola-Jurado N, Basora J, et al. Reduction in the incidence of type 2 diabetes with the Mediterranean diet: results of the PREDIMED-Reus Nutrition Intervention Randomized Trial. Diabetes Care 2010 Oct 13.

48. Lindstrom J, Neumann A, Sheppard KE, Gilis-Januszewska A, Greaves CJ, Handke U, et al. Take action to prevent diabetes: the IMAGE toolkit for the prevention of type 2 diabetes in Europe. Horm Metab Res 2010;42(Suppl 1):S37–55.

CHAPTER 2

Identification of target populations for intervention

Paul Valensi and Emmanuel Cosson

Department of Endocrinology Diabetology Nutrition, Jean Verdier Hospital, AP-HP, Paris Nord University, CRNH-IdF, Bondy, France

Introduction

The increasing prevalence of diabetes highlights the role of several risk factors. The development of type 2 diabetes (T2D) results from a complex interplay between genetic and environmental factors. A large number of individuals have undiagnosed glucose abnormalities. The accurate evaluation of the risk for diabetes helps in identifying the target populations for preventive actions to reverse the global progression of T2D.

Risk factors for type 2 diabetes

The risk for T2D is determined by the cumulative influence of the number and severity of nonmodifiable and modifiable risk factors.

Nonmodifiable risk factors

Age is one of the strongest risk factors for T2D. In European populations mean 2-h plasma glucose concentration after an oral 75-g glucose load (OGTT) increases linearly with age while fasting plasma glucose concentration does not. The prevalence of diabetes rises up to the eighth decade [1].

Evidence for a genetic component in the pathogenesis of T2D comes from twin studies. The risk of T2D increases more than twofold if a first-degree relative is affected [2]. At least 25 gene loci that increase the risk for T2D have been identified [3]. Most of these genes have a role in beta-cell

Prevention of Diabetes, First Edition. Edited by Peter Schwarz and Prasuna Reddy.
© 2013 John Wiley & Sons, Ltd. Published 2013 by John Wiley & Sons, Ltd.

function rather than in insulin sensitivity. However, these variants explain less than 10% of the genetic basis of diabetes risk. Therefore it is still too early to use genetic data for targeting preventive strategies.

Some ethnic groups have a genetic predisposition to develop diabetes. According to the "thrifty gene" hypothesis, various genetic defects or poly-morphisms could contribute to diabetes when people are exposed to increased food availability. The prevalence of diabetes in Hispanics is 1.9 times higher than in Caucasians [4]. Afro-Caribbeans and Asian Indians also have a high prevalence of T2D [5].

Women with a history of gestational diabetes mellitus (GDM) have an approximately 7.5-fold increased risk for T2D compared with women with normoglycemic pregnancy [6]. Maternal age greater than 40 years, high OGTT 2-h values during pregnancy, and insulin treatment during preg-nancy were reported to predict impaired glucose tolerance (IGT) in women 1 year postpartum following GDM [7].

Most women with polycystic ovary syndrome (PCOS) have increased insulin resistance and impaired beta-cell function even in the absence of clinically evident glucose intolerance [8]. Around 30% of women with PCOS have IGT and up to 10% are diabetic [9]. A recent meta-analysis reported an approximately threefold increased risk of GDM among women with PCOS [10].

Modifiable risk factors

Obesity and overweight increase the risk of developing both IGT and T2D, at least partially by inducing insulin resistance. A curvilinear relationship between body mass index (BMI) and the risk of T2D was found in women in the Nurses' Health Study [11]. In addition to the degree of obesity, the distribution of excess fat is an important determinant of the risk of insulin resistance and T2D.

A meta-analysis demonstrated a U-shaped relationship between birth weight and diabetes risk [12]. Subjects who had a low birth weight for gestational age, as adults had reduced beta-cell function, insulin resistance, and a greater incidence of T2D. Fetal malnutrition can also result in changes leading to less efficient substrate utilization, a process that can be imprinted during pregnancy. Future exposure to abundance of calories may contribute to central obesity and insulin resistance. Higher birth weight (>4 kg) is also associated with an increased risk for T2D. Children born prematurely may also be at increased risk for T2D and other diseases of adulthood associated with insulin resistance [13].

Impaired fasting glucose (IFG) and IGT are early abnormalities of glucose metabolism that precede diabetes and are often termed prediabetes. IFG is defined by the International Diabetes Federation (IDF) as an elevated fasting plasma glucose (FPG) concentration (110–126 mg/dL). In 2003 the cutoff value for IFG was changed to 100 mg/dL by the American Diabetes Association (ADA). IGT is defined as an elevated 2-h plasma glucose concentration (140–200 mg/dL) during OGTT, in the presence of an FPG concentration <126 mg/dL [14,15]. IFG and IGT can be isolated or associated. Some studies suggest that IGT is primarily associated with insulin resistance and IFG with impaired insulin secretion and suppression of hepatic glucose output. The prevalence of IFG and IGT vary across ethnic groups and is positively associated with age. In a recent meta-analysis, the relative risk for progression to diabetes was 6.35 for people with IGT, 4.66 for people with IFG, and 12.13 for those with IFG and IGT [16]. It can be estimated that over a period of 3–5 years about 25% of individuals with such prediabetic disorders progress to diabetes [17].

The metabolic syndrome (MetS) is defined as a cluster of metabolic risk factors for cardiovascular disease (CVD) that are associated with insulin resistance. The most widely used definition for MetS is the one issued by the third report of the National Cholesterol Education Program Expert Panel on detection, evaluation, and treatment of high blood cholesterol in adults, and includes central obesity, high FPG, high plasma triglycerides, low plasma high-density lipoprotein (HDL) cholesterol, and high blood pressure [18]. Another definition has recently been suggested in a joint statement from several international organizations [19]. The presence of MetS is associated with a higher risk of T2D [20]. However, a single measure of blood glucose appeared to be a better predictor of incident diabetes than MetS [21], although in the San Antonio heart study, MetS predicted T2D better than fasting glucose values [22].

Dietary factors are considered to have an important role in the development of diabetes. Diet can act by changing body weight. However, although several confounding factors limit the conclusions from nutritional studies, some specific dietary factors can predict T2D. Fiber has a low glycemic index, which may contribute to reducing the risk of T2D. A recent meta-analysis showed that both high glycemic load and high glycemic index diets were associated with increased risk for T2D [23]. Switching from a diet based on animal fat to a diet richer in vegetable fat could reduce this risk. An increased intake of monounsaturated fat may also be beneficial [24]. However, trans fatty acids consumption was shown to be associated with increased risk. Consumption of moderate amounts of alcohol, fruits and vegetables, fish and nuts are suggested to reduce the risk. A dietary pattern like the "Mediterranean diet" was shown to be associated with a reduced risk of diabetes [25].

A recent meta-analysis of 10 prospective cohort studies reported a lower risk of developing diabetes with regular moderate physical activity compared with being sedentary [26]. The benefit of exercise in preventing diabetes has been demonstrated in several studies.

Psychosocial factors may have a causal role in the events leading to MetS [27]. An increased risk of developing T2D in depressed adults has been demonstrated in a recent meta-analysis [28].

An inverse association has consistently been reported between socioeconomic status and T2D, across several developed countries and different ethnic groups, with a higher prevalence among less advantaged groups.

A long list of drugs can impair glucose tolerance by decreasing insulin secretion, increasing hepatic glucose production, or causing resistance to the action of insulin [29].

Target populations for intervention

The IDF consensus [30] recommends population-based as well as individually targeted approaches for diabetes prevention.

Population approach

This approach should be based on environmental conditions able to favor the achievement and maintenance of a healthy lifestyle. National diabetes prevention plans are required. As an example, a study performed in the United Kingdom suggests encouraging the achievement of five healthy behavior goals including BMI $<25\,kg/m^2$, fat intake $<30\%$ of energy intake, saturated fat intake $<10\%$ of energy intake, fiber intake $\geq15\,g/4184\,kJ$, and physical activity >4 hour/week in order to reduce the incidence of diabetes [31].

High-risk approach

In several countries, targeted or opportunistic screening to identify high-risk individuals is recommended in current practice. The IDF consensus [30] recommends opportunistic screening by health care providers using the following criteria: obesity, family history of diabetes, age, history of hypertension and/or heart disease, GDM history, and drug history. Risk for T2D and CVD may be assessed quantitatively by appropriate methods such as blood testing and searching for the presence of other risk factors. Appropriate interventions targeting all identified risk factors should subsequently be initiated.

Hierarchical approach for intervention

Individuals with IGT are at highest risk for T2D, but those with isolated IFG and MetS also have an increased risk. Particularly high mean annual conversion rates (>10%) have been reported in subjects combining two or three prediabetic conditions (IGT ± IFG, ± MetS) [22,32]. Therefore, because of limited resources, a hierarchical approach aiming to provide the most intensive intervention to the highest risk subjects has been proposed in the IMAGE project [33], starting with subjects with IGT ± IFG (± MetS) with highest priority, followed by subjects with IFG and/or MetS with high priority, subjects with overweight, obesity, hypertension, or physical inactivity with medium priority, and finally the general population with low priority.

Categorization of glucose abnormalities

Glucometabolic category depends on whether plasma glucose is measured only at fasting or also after an oral glucose load (OGTT).

According to epidemiologic studies, a large number of subjects who do not meet the FPG criteria for glucose disorders will satisfy the criteria when exposed to an OGTT [1,34]. Thus, the OGTT is more sensitive than FPG for detecting diabetes and is the only way to detect IGT. However, there are some arguments against OGTT. This test should be standardized and carried out after at least 3 days of unrestricted carbohydrate diet. OGTT has been considered to be less appropriate at a population level, mainly because it is time consuming, costly, and has low reproducibility. However, because prevention of diabetes needs to identify high-risk subjects, a definite categorization of glycemic status is mandatory. It must be pointed out that most of the prevention trials included patients with IGT. In addition, patients with IGT are also at high risk for developing CVD. Many individuals with prediabetes have a clustering of other cardiovascular risk factors, and a number of subjects with IGT will develop CVD before progressing to diabetes.

For all these reasons, it is strongly suggested that clinicians categorize the type of glycemic abnormalities as precisely as possible, identify people with IGT, and screen those with IGT for associated CVD risk factors in order to achieve the goals of both diabetes and CVD prevention. However, this step should be applied after a screening phase able to identify subjects with a high a priori chance of detecting prediabetes or diabetes.

Detection of people at high risk for diabetes: scoring systems

Combining all the risk factors for diabetes and weighting their impact appears logical and appealing. A number of scores have been developed to screen for the risk of incident (Table 2.1) or undiagnosed diabetes (Table 2.2) including clinical, biologic, or genetic parameters. However, the clinical scores are the most used as they are cheap, simple, and practical. Furthermore, adding biologic parameters often does not improve the screening performance, except for the measurement of plasma glucose. Scores can be used routinely by the individual who wishes to know his/her own risk. We here overview questionnaires that have been developed in Europe (FINDRISK), the United States (ADA diabetes risk score), and Asia.

The Finnish risk test (FINDRISK) comprises eight scored questions, with the total test score providing a measure of the probability of developing T2D over the following 10 years. This test takes only a couple of minutes to complete. Seven variables clearly correlated with the risk of developing diabetes were chosen: age, BMI, waist circumference, use of antihypertensive medication, history of elevated blood glucose (which includes previous GDM), daily physical activity, and daily intake of fruit or vegetables. The variables were assigned scores according to the relative risk conferred by each one in a logistic regression model, yielding a range of 0–20 for the total score. Physical activity and fruit and vegetable consumption were kept in the score to increase awareness about the importance of lifestyle modifications, even if they were not associated with a much elevated diabetes risk. The more points scored in the test, the higher the risk of incident diabetes.

A limitation to the study was that only drug-treated diabetes was considered as incident outcome. However, a score value ≥9 had sensitivity of 0.78, specificity of 0.77, and positive predictive value of 0.13. The score was validated for incident diabetes in an independent population survey performed in 1992 with prospective follow-up for 5 years [35], and also in Germany [36] and France [37]. On the basis of other studies, family

Table 2.1 Methods to screen for incident dysglycemia.

Data source/follow-up time (reference)	Age (years)	n	Dysglycemia diagnosis	Predictive variables	Area under the receiver-operating characteristic curve
San Antonio Heart Study (7.5 years) [17]	25–64	2903	Diabetes (OGTT or medical records)	Clinical model: age, sex, ethnicity, fasting glucose, systolic blood pressure, HDL cholesterol, body mass index, family history of diabetes	0.84
				Full model: also 2-h glucose, diastolic blood pressure, total and LDL cholesterol, triglyceride	0.86
Rancho Bernardo Study [68]	67 ± 11	1549	Impaired glucose tolerance	Sex, age, triglycerides, fasting glucose	
Model validation: Health ABC Study (5 years)	70–79	2503	Diabetes (medical records)		0.71
Atherosclerosis Risk in Communities Study (9 years) [69]	45–64	7915	Diabetes (OGTT or medical records)	Model 1: age, ethnicity, waist, height, fasting glucose, systolic blood pressure, family history of diabetes	0.78
				Model 2: also HDL cholesterol and triglycerides	0.80
Finnish Diabetes Risk Score (FINDRISK) (10 years) [35]	35–64	4435	Antidiabetic treatment	Age, body mass index, waist circumference, use of antihypertensive therapy, history of high blood glucose	0.85
Model validation	45–64	4615	Antidiabetic treatment		0.87
Data from the Epidemiologic Study on the Insulin Resistance syndrome (DESIR) (9 years) [37]	30–65	3817	Fasting plasma glucose ≥7 mmol	Clinical model: waist circumference, hypertension and smoking (men) or familial history of diabetes (women)	0.71 (men) 0.83 (women)
Model validation: SU.VI.MAX			Fasting plasma glucose ≥7 mmol or treatment		0.85
Model validation: E3N			Self question treatment		0.92

HDL, high-density lipoprotein; LDL, low-density lipoprotein; OGTT, oral glucose tolerance test.

Table 2.2 Methods to screen for prevalent type 2 diabetes.

Data source	Age (years)	n	Diabetes diagnosis	Predictive variables	Area under the receiver-operating characteristic curve
"The ADA risk score" Second National Health and Nutrition Examination Survey [42]	20–74	3770	OGTT	Age, sex, delivery of macrosomic infant, race, education, obesity, sedentary lifestyle, family history of diabetes	0.78
Rotterdam Predictive Model [51]	55–75	1016	OGTT	Model 1: age, sex, presence of obesity, use of antihypertensive medication Model 2: + family history of diabetes, physical inactivity, body mass index	Model 1: 0.68 Model 2: 0.74
Model validation: Hoorn Study	50–74	2364			
The Cambridge risk score [70] Model development: * Ely Study (ES), Wessex Study (WS)	40–64	650	ES: OGTT, WS: diabetes diagnosed during 12 months	Age, sex, body mass index, family history of diabetes, use of antihypertensive or steroid medication, smoking	
Model validation: ** Ely Study [71]	40–64 39–78	528 6567	HbA1c ≥7%		0.80 0.74
Inter99 Model development: * Inter99 [72]	30–60	3250	OGTT	Age, sex, body mass index, family history of diabetes, known hypertension, physical activity	0.80
Model validation: ** Inter99	30–60	2874			0.76
ADDITION pilot study	40–69	1028			0.80

* First half and ** second half of the study population.

history of diabetes was incorporated in the final test, which made the maximum score 26. Afterwards, the score was shown to be associated with current undiagnosed T2D, prediabetic states, MetS, and cardiovascular risk factors in a Finnish [38], Italian [39], Greek [40] and also a French cohort of women with overweight or obesity [41]. In conclusion, the FINDRISK score successfully addresses the required conditions to be a simple, non-invasive, and inexpensive tool in Europe, with a double perspective: detecting undiagnosed diabetes and predicting incident diabetes.

The ADA risk score includes only clinical parameters (Table 2.2) [42]. The score derived from the San Antonio Heart Study also includes FPG and HDL cholesterol but does not perform better than FPG alone [17].

Scores from Asia have shown similar performances, and use the same parameters to predict incident diabetes or prevalent dysglycemia. The Indian Diabetes Risk Score for undiagnosed diabetes has been developed from the Chennai Urban Rural Epidemiological Study (CURES). This simple test, which includes four factors (age, waist circumference, family history of diabetes, and physical activity), has an optimum sensitivity of 72% and specificity of 60%, with a positive predictive value of 17% and a negative predictive value of 95% [43]. A simple risk equation (including age, BMI, and hypertension) has also been defined in a high-risk Thai population and has been shown to detect 87% of undiagnosed diabetes [44]. Three recent Chinese scores have been reported to predict prevalent diabetes [45,46] or an abnormal OGTT [47], considering simple clinical parameters as age, gender, BMI, hypertension, dyslipidemia, family history of diabetes and GDM [46], or waist circumference, age, and family history of diabetes [45]. Liu et al. [47] showed that the association of clinical and biologic parameters predicted both prevalent and incident diabetes in Chinese cohorts.

The scoring systems have some limits:

1 Screening tests using questionnaires need to be performed in appropriate conditions. The FINDRISK may be used as a self-administered test. However, it is recommended that the answers should be checked by a nurse or a physician.

2 More importantly, the performances of the scores are not similar worldwide. For example, four published screening tests (Rotterdam Diabetes Study, Cambridge Risk score, San Antonio Heart Study, and FINDRISK), when applied in a German population (KORA Survey 2000) to detect undiagnosed diabetes, yielded low validity, most likely because of differences in population characteristics [48]. The performance of FINDRISK to detect current glycemic status was also found to be low

in German subjects with a family history of T2D [36] and in the population of Oman [49]. The DETECT-2 project, an international data pooling collaboration specifically addressed issues related to screening for T2D, with an emphasis on the impact of ethnicity and population differences on screening protocols [50]. Nine datasets representative of people from a diverse range of ethnic backgrounds (northern and southern Europe, United States, Indian subcontinent, Asia, Australia, Pacific Islands, and Africa) were selected. The performances of the Rotterdam Predictive Model [51] varied widely, with sensitivity, specificity, and percentage needing further testing ranging 12–57%, 72–93%, and 2–25%, respectively, with the worse performance in non-Caucasian populations.

3 The thresholds for variables such as BMI or waist circumference have to be adapted for Asian people [45–47]. This suggests that performance of diabetes risk questionnaires or scores must be assessed in the target population where they will be ultimately applied.

However, all these screening tools have a high negative predictive value (94–98%), and thus may be helpful when the findings are negative rather than positive.

After scoring for diabetes risk, it is mandatory to inform those patients with elevated risk.

Strategies to identify people at high risk for diabetes

Community-based strategies

Various approaches are possible:

1 Measuring plasma glucose to determine prevalent prediabetes, a strategy that will also detect undiagnosed diabetes.

2 Collecting questionnaires that provide an estimate of the risk for incident diabetes, a strategy that leaves the current glycemic state undetermined.

3 Collecting questionnaires as primary screening tools, and identifying a subgroup of the population in whom glycemic testing may be targeted efficiently at baseline and follow-up.

The last alternative has been tested in the IGLOO study [39]. FINDRISK was evaluated as a first step, then FPG was measured in individuals with a score ≥9. Finally, OGTT was performed when FPG was 5.6–6.9 mmol/L. This strategy identified 83% of the subjects with T2D and 57% of those with IGT, whereas FPG measurement and OGTT would have been performed in 64% and 38% of the sample, respectively [39].

In agreement with the IDF [30], the use of opportunistic screening by health care personnel (including those working in general practice, nurses, and pharmacists) or by anyone on the Internet and secondarily validated by a health care provider, was recently recommended by the IMAGE project consortium [33]. After step 1, a person considered to be at increased risk for diabetes will proceed to the measurement of plasma glucose at fasting or, even better, during an OGTT in order to determine their glycemic state more precisely. This second step depends on the resources available. At the very least, measurement of random capillary blood glucose can be used with an improved performance if measurement is carried out in the postprandial period [52].

Clinical practice-based strategies

A screening test may be used in routine clinical practice but, as it is time consuming, it is suggested to select patients with at least one obvious risk factor for diabetes. Several criteria have been proposed [30,53]. Those from the IMAGE project consortium are summarized in Table 2.3.

Table 2.3 Criteria for screening for diabetes within targeted populations [33].

1. White people aged over 40 years and people from black, Asian and minority ethnic groups aged over 25 with one or more of the risk factors below:
   - a first-degree family history of diabetes, and/or
   - BMI >25 kg/m², and/or
   - waist measurement of ≥94 cm for white and black men and ≥ 80 cm for white, black and Asian women, and ≥90 cm for Asian men, and/or
   - systolic blood pressure ≥140 mmHg or diastolic blood pressure ≥90 mmHg or treated hypertension, and/or
   - HDL cholesterol ≤35 mg/dL (0.9 mmol) or triglycerides ≥200 mg/dL (2.2 mmol) or treated dyslipidemia
2. History of gestational diabetes or child with birth weight >4 kg
3. History of temporarily induced diabetes
4. People who have ischemic heart disease, cerebrovascular disease, or peripheral vascular disease
5. Women with polycystic ovary syndrome who have a BMI ≥30 kg/m²
6. People who have severe mental health problems and/or receiving long-term antipsychotic drugs
7. History of IGT or IFG

BMI, body mass index; HDL, high density lipoprotein; IFT, impaired fasting glucose; IGT, impaired glucose tolerance.

An OGTT should always be performed in some populations: women with previous GDM and patients having experienced an acute coronary syndrome. The sensitivity of FPG compared with OGTT is poor in women with a history of GDM, at 16–89% [54–57]. Furthermore, OGTT every 3 years compared with FPG measurement offers a lower cost per T2D diagnosis in this population [58].

Patients without known diabetes and who experience an acute coronary syndrome (ACS) have a very high prevalence of abnormal glucose metabolism at discharge [59], 2 [60], 3 [59] and 12 months thereafter [61]: about one-third have diabetes and one-third have prediabetes. The prevalence was reported to be almost twice as common amongst patients with ACS than in matched controls [62]. The prevalence was also very high in a series of patients referred for coronary angiography [63] or for elective cardiology[60]. As reported in subjects without ACS [64], OGTT is needed for appropriate classification of glucose status. Very consistently, performing only FPG measurement leads to underdiagnosing dysglycemic states in two-thirds of ACS patients [59,62]. This is also true when applying 5.5 rather than 6.0 mmol/L as the FPG threshold to define IFG [65]. According to a recent French consensus statement, patients with HbA1c ≥6.5% on admission for an ACS may be considered diabetic while, in those with no known diabetes and HbA1c <6.5%, it is recommended that an OGTT be performed 7–28 days after ACS [66].

The sensitivity of FPG to diagnose dysglycemia compared with OGTT is also poor in patients with overweight or obesity: 33.3 and 29.9% for the diagnosis of diabetes and dysglycemia, respectively [67]. However, performing an OGTT to diagnose dysglycemia in all subjects with overweight or obesity appears to be inconvenient and time consuming. The authors recently tested strategies using OGTT only in obese women with a high clinical score or a high HbA1c [41]. Thresholds maximizing sensitivity and specificity were 4 points for DESIR score and a new simple score (Bondy score, using only waist circumference and age), 12 points for FINDRISK, and 5.7% for HbA1c. Overall, these strategies led to limit OGTT to 40–60% of the cohort, with a sensitivity of 60–75%, whereas measuring only FPG in all women had a sensitivity of 27% to diagnose dysglycemia. This strategy also appeared to be cost effective using the scores but not HbA1c [41].

Conclusions

It is of major importance in at-risk subjects to define glycemic status in order to diagnose and manage T2D earlier and to detect earlier those with

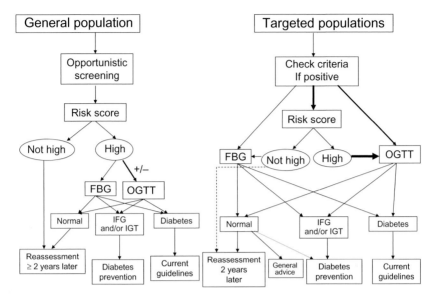

Figure 2.1 Screening strategy for diabetes and prediabetes [33]. FBG, fasting blood glucose; IFG, impaired fasting glucose; IGT, impaired glucose tolerance; OGTT, oral glucose tolerance test.

prediabetes who would benefit from preventive actions. The screening strategy for identifying diabetes and prediabetes in the general population and in targeted populations can be based on an algorithm (Figure 2.1) which includes the use of a scoring system and glucose measurement.

References

1. Decode Study Group. Age- and sex-specific prevalences of diabetes and impaired glucose regulation in 13 European cohorts. Diabetes Care 2003;26:61–9.
2. Lyssenko V, Almgren P, Anevski D, Perfekt R, Lahti K, Nissén M, et al. Predictors of and longitudinal changes in insulin sensitivity and secretion preceding onset of type 2 diabetes. Diabetes 2005;54:166–74.
3. Stolerman ES,Florez JC. Genomics of type 2 diabetes mellitus: implications for the clinician. Nat Rev Endocrinol 2009;5:429–36.
4. Umpierrez GE, Gonzalez A, Umpierrez D, Pimentel D. Diabetes mellitus in the Hispanic/Latino population: an increasing health care challenge in the United States. Am J Med Sci 2007;334:274–82.
5. Davis TM. Ethnic diversity in type 2 diabetes. Diabet Med 2008;25 Suppl 2:52–6.
6. Bellamy L, Casas JP, Hingorani AD, Williams D. Type 2 diabetes mellitus after gestational diabetes: a systematic review and meta-analysis. Lancet 2009;373:1773–9.

7. Aberg AE, Jonsson EK, Eskilsson I, Landin-Olsson M, Frid AH. Predictive factors of developing diabetes mellitus in women with gestational diabetes. Acta Obstet Gynecol Scand 2002;81:11–6.

8. Dabadghao P, Roberts BJ, Wang J, Davies MJ, Norman RJ. Glucose tolerance abnormalities in Australian women with polycystic ovary syndrome. Med J Aust 2007; 187:328–31.

9. Ehrmann DA, Barnes RB, Rosenfield RL, Cavaghan MK, Imperial J. Prevalence of impaired glucose tolerance and diabetes in women with polycystic ovary syndrome. Diabetes Care 1999;22:141–6.

10. Boomsma CM, Eijkemans MJ, Hughes EG, Visser GH, Fauser BC, Macklon NS. A meta-analysis of pregnancy outcomes in women with polycystic ovary syndrome. Hum Reprod Update 2006;12:673–83.

11. Colditz GA, Willett WC, Rotnitzky A, Manson JE. Weight gain as a risk factor for clinical diabetes mellitus in women. Ann Intern Med 1995;122:481–6.

12. Harder T, Rodekamp E, Schellong K, Dudenhausen JW, Plagemann A. Birth weight and subsequent risk of type 2 diabetes: a meta-analysis. Am J Epidemiol 2007;165: 849–57.

13. Hofman PL, Regan F, Jackson WE, Jefferies C, Knight DB, Robinson EM, et al. Premature birth and later insulin resistance. N Engl J Med 2004;351:2179–86.

14. Genuth S, Alberti KG, Bennett P, Buse J, Defronzo R, Kahn R, et al. Follow-up report on the diagnosis of diabetes mellitus. Diabetes Care 2003;26:3160–7.

15. Alberti KG, Zimmet PZ. Definition, diagnosis and classification of diabetes mellitus and its complications. Part 1: diagnosis and classification of diabetes mellitus provisional report of a WHO consultation. Diabet Med 1998;15:539–53.

16. Gerstein HC, Santaguida P, Raina P, Morrison KM, Balion C, Hunt D, et al. Annual incidence and relative risk of diabetes in people with various categories of dysglycemia: a systematic overview and meta-analysis of prospective studies. Diabetes Res Clin Pract 2007;78:305–12.

17. Stern MP, Williams K, Haffner SM. Identification of persons at high risk for type 2 diabetes mellitus: do we need the oral glucose tolerance test? Ann Intern Med 2002;136:575–81.

18. Third Report of the National Cholesterol Education Program (NCEP) Expert Panel on Detection, Evaluation, and Treatment of High Blood Cholesterol in Adults (Adult Treatment Panel III) final report. Circulation 2002;106:3143–421.

19. Alberti KG, Eckel RH, Grundy SM, Zimmet PZ, Cleeman JI, Donato KA, et al. Harmonizing the metabolic syndrome: a joint interim statement of the International Diabetes Federation Task Force on Epidemiology and Prevention; National Heart, Lung, and Blood Institute; American Heart Association; World Heart Federation; International Atherosclerosis Society; and International Association for the Study of Obesity. Circulation 2009;120:1640–5.

20. Ford ES, Li C, Sattar N. Metabolic syndrome and incident diabetes: current state of the evidence. Diabetes Care 2008;31:1898–904.

21. Hanley AJ, Karter AJ, Williams K, Festa A, D'Agostino RB Jr, Wagenknecht LE, et al. Prediction of type 2 diabetes mellitus with alternative definitions of the metabolic syndrome: the Insulin Resistance Atherosclerosis Study. Circulation 2005;112: 3713–21.

22. Lorenzo C, Williams K, Hunt KJ, Haffner SM. The National Cholesterol Education Program: Adult Treatment Panel III, International Diabetes Federation, and World

Health Organization definitions of the metabolic syndrome as predictors of incident cardiovascular disease and diabetes. Diabetes Care 2007;30:8–13.

23. Barclay AW, Petocz P, McMillan-Price J, Flood VM, Prvan T, Mitchell P, et al. Glycemic index, glycemic load, and chronic disease risk: a meta-analysis of observational studies. Am J Clin Nutr 2008;87:627–37.

24. Due A, Larsen TM, Hermansen K, Stender S, Holst JJ, Toubro S, et al. Comparison of the effects on insulin resistance and glucose tolerance of 6-mo high-monounsaturated-fat, low-fat, and control diets. Am J Clin Nutr 2008;87:855–62.

25. Martinez-Gonzalez MA, de la Fuente-Arrillaga C, Nunez-Cordoba JM, Basterra-Gortari FJ, Beunza JJ, Vazquez Z, et al. Adherence to Mediterranean diet and risk of developing diabetes: prospective cohort study. BMJ 2008;336:1348–51.

26. Jeon CY, Lokken RP, Hu FB, van Dam RM. Physical activity of moderate intensity and risk of type 2 diabetes: a systematic review. Diabetes Care 2007;30:744–52.

27. La Rosa E, Le Clesiau H,Valensi P. Metabolic syndrome and psychosocial deprivation. Data collected from a Paris suburb. Diabetes Metab 2008;34:155–61.

28. Knol MJ, Twisk JW, Beekman AT, Heine RJ, Snoek FJ, Pouwer F. Depression as a risk factor for the onset of type 2 diabetes mellitus: a meta-analysis. Diabetologia 2006;49:837–45.

29. Luna B, Feinglos MN. Drug-induced hyperglycemia. JAMA 2001;286:1945–8.

30. Alberti KG, Zimmet P, Shaw J. International Diabetes Federation: a consensus on type 2 diabetes prevention. Diabet Med 2007;24:451–63.

31. Simmons RK, Harding AH, Jakes RW, Welch A, Wareham NJ, Griffin SJ. How much might achievement of diabetes prevention behaviour goals reduce the incidence of diabetes if implemented at the population level? Diabetologia 2006;49:905–11.

32. de Vegt F, Dekker JM, Jager A, Hienkens E, Kostense PJ, Stehouwer CD, et al. Relation of impaired fasting and postload glucose with incident type 2 diabetes in a Dutch population: The Hoorn Study. JAMA 2001;285:2109–13.

33. Paulweber B, Valensi P, Lindstrom J, Lalic NM, Greaves CJ, McKee M, et al. A European evidence-based guideline for the prevention of type 2 diabetes. Horm Metab Res 2010;42(Suppl 1):S3–36.

34. Qiao Q, Hu G, Tuomilehto J, Nakagami T, Balkau B, Borch-Johnsen K, et al. Age- and sex-specific prevalence of diabetes and impaired glucose regulation in 11 Asian cohorts. Diabetes Care 2003;26:1770–80.

35. Lindstrom J, Tuomilehto J. The diabetes risk score: a practical tool to predict type 2 diabetes risk. Diabetes Care 2003;26:725–31.

36. Bergmann A, Li J, Wang L, Bornstein SR, Schwarz PE. A simplified Finnish diabetes risk score to predict type 2 diabetes risk and disease evolution in a German population. Horm Metab Res 2007;39:677–82.

37. Balkau B, Lange C, Fezeu L, Tichet J, de Lauzon-Guillain B, Czernichow S, et al. Predicting diabetes: clinical, biological, and genetic approaches: data from the Epidemiological Study on the Insulin Resistance Syndrome (DESIR). Diabetes Care 2008;31:2056–61.

38. Saaristo T, Peltonen M, Lindstrom J, Saarikoski L, Sundvall J, Eriksson JG, et al. Cross-sectional evaluation of the Finnish Diabetes Risk Score: a tool to identify undetected type 2 diabetes, abnormal glucose tolerance and metabolic syndrome. Diab Vasc Dis Res 2005;2:67–72.

39. Franciosi M, De Berardis G, Rossi MC, Sacco M, Belfiglio M, Pellegrini F, et al. Use of the diabetes risk score for opportunistic screening of undiagnosed diabetes and

impaired glucose tolerance: the IGLOO (Impaired Glucose Tolerance and Long-Term Outcomes Observational) study. Diabetes Care 2005;28:1187–94.

40. Makrilakis K, Liatis S, Grammatikou S, Perrea D, Stathi C, Tsiligros P, et al. Validation of the Finnish diabetes risk score (FINDRISC) questionnaire for screening for undiagnosed type 2 diabetes, dysglycaemia and the metabolic syndrome in Greece. Diabetes Metab 2011;37:144–51.

41. Cosson E, Chiheb S, Hamo-Tchatchouang E, Nguyen MT, Aout M, Banu I, et al. Use of clinical scores to detect dysglycemia in overweight or obese women. Diabetes Metab 2012;38:217–224.

42. Herman WH, Smith PJ, Thompson TJ, Engelgau MM, Aubert RE. A new and simple questionnaire to identify people at increased risk for undiagnosed diabetes. Diabetes Care 1995;18:382–7.

43. Mohan V, Deepa R, Deepa M, Somannavar S, Datta M. A simplified Indian Diabetes Risk Score for screening for undiagnosed diabetic subjects. J Assoc Physicians India 2005;53:759–63.

44. Keesukphan P, Chanprasertyothin S, Ongphiphadhanakul B, Puavilai G. The development and validation of a diabetes risk score for high-risk Thai adults. J Med Assoc Thai 2007;90:149–54.

45. Gao WG, Dong YH, Pang ZC, Nan HR, Wang SJ, Ren J, et al. A simple Chinese risk score for undiagnosed diabetes. Diabet Med 2010;27:274–81.

46. Ko G, So W, Tong P, Ma R, Kong A, Ozaki R, et al. A simple risk score to identify Southern Chinese at high risk for diabetes. Diabet Med 2010;27:644–9.

47. Liu M, Pan C, Jin M. A Chinese diabetes risk score for screening of undiagnosed diabetes and abnormal glucose tolerance. Diabetes Technol Ther 2011;13:501–7.

48. Rathmann W, Martin S, Haastert B, Icks A, Holle R, Löwel H, et al. Performance of screening questionnaires and risk scores for undiagnosed diabetes: the KORA Survey 2000. Arch Intern Med 2005;165:436–41.

49. Al-Lawati JA, Tuomilehto J. Diabetes risk score in Oman: a tool to identify prevalent type 2 diabetes among Arabs of the Middle East. Diabetes Res Clin Pract 2007;77: 438–44.

50. Glumer C, Vistisen D, Borch-Johnsen K, Colagiuri S; DETECT-2 Collaboration. Risk scores for type 2 diabetes can be applied in some populations but not all. Diabetes Care 2006;29:410–4.

51. Baan CA, Ruige JB, Stolk RP, Witteman JC, Dekker JM, Heine RJ, et al. Performance of a predictive model to identify undiagnosed diabetes in a health care setting. Diabetes Care 1999;22:213–9.

52. Engelgau MM, Thompson TJ, Smith PJ, Herman WH, Aubert RE, Gunter EW, et al. Screening for diabetes mellitus in adults: the utility of random capillary blood glucose measurements. Diabetes Care 1995;18:463–6.

53. ADA. Clinical practice recommendations 2008. Diabetes Care 2008;31:S1–S110.

54. Bennett WL, Bolen S, Wilson LM, Bass EB, Nicholson WK. Performance characteristics of postpartum screening tests for type 2 diabetes mellitus in women with a history of gestational diabetes mellitus: a systematic review. J Womens Health (Larchmt) 2009;18:979–87.

55. Kwong S, Mitchell RS, Senior PA, Chik CL. Postpartum diabetes screening: adherence rate and the performance of fasting plasma glucose versus oral glucose tolerance test. Diabetes Care 2009;32:2242–4.

56. Ferrara A, Peng T, Kim C. Trends in postpartum diabetes screening and subsequent diabetes and impaired fasting glucose among women with histories of gestational diabetes mellitus: a report from the Translating Research Into Action for Diabetes (TRIAD) Study. Diabetes Care 2009;32:269–74.

57. Flack JR, Payne TJ,Ross GP. Post-partum glucose tolerance assessment in women diagnosed with gestational diabetes: evidence supporting the need to undertake an oral glucose tolerance test. Diabet Med 2010;27:243–4.

58. Kim C, Herman WH, Vijan S. Efficacy and cost of postpartum screening strategies for diabetes among women with histories of gestational diabetes mellitus. Diabetes Care 2007;30:1102–6.

59. Norhammar A, Tenerz A, Nilsson G, Hamsten A, Efendíc S, Rydén L, et al. Glucose metabolism in patients with acute myocardial infarction and no previous diagnosis of diabetes mellitus: a prospective study. Lancet 2002;359:2140–4.

60. Bartnik M, Rydén L, Ferrari R, Malmberg K, Pyörälä K, Simoons M, et al. The prevalence of abnormal glucose regulation in patients with coronary artery disease across Europe. The Euro Heart Survey on diabetes and the heart. Eur Heart J 2004;25:1880–90.

61. Wallander M, Malmberg K, Norhammar A, Rydén L, Tenerz A. Oral glucose tolerance test: a reliable tool for early detection of glucose abnormalities in patients with acute myocardial infarction in clinical practice: a report on repeated oral glucose tolerance tests from the GAMI study. Diabetes Care 2008;31:36–8.

62. Bartnik M, Malmberg K, Hamsten A, Efendic S, Norhammar A, Silveira A, et al. Abnormal glucose tolerance: a common risk factor in patients with acute myocardial infarction in comparison with population-based controls. J Intern Med 2004; 256:288–97.

63. Kowalska I, Prokop J, Bachórzewska-Gajewska H, Telejko B, Kinalskal I, Kochman W, et al. Disturbances of glucose metabolism in men referred for coronary arteriography: postload glycemia as predictor for coronary atherosclerosis. Diabetes Care 2001;24:897–901.

64. Is fasting glucose sufficient to define diabetes? Epidemiological data from 20 European studies. The DECODE-study group. European Diabetes Epidemiology Group. Diabetes Epidemiology: Collaborative analysis of Diagnostic Criteria in Europe. Diabetologia 1999;42:647–54.

65. Bartnik M, Rydén L, Malmberg K, Ohrvik J, Pyörälä K, Standl E, et al. Oral glucose tolerance test is needed for appropriate classification of glucose regulation in patients with coronary artery disease: a report from the Euro Heart Survey on Diabetes and the Heart. Heart 2007;93:72–7.

66. Vergès B, Avignon A, Bonnet F, Catargi B, Cattan S, Cosson E, et al. Consensus statement on the care of the hyperglycaemic/diabetic patient during and in the immediate follow-up of acute coronary syndrome. Diabetes Metab 2012;38:113–27.

67. Cosson E, Hamo-Tchatchouang E, Banu I, Nguyen MT, Chiheb S, Ba H, et al. A large proportion of prediabetes and diabetes goes undiagnosed when only fasting plasma glucose and/or HbA1c are measured in overweight or obese patients. Diabetes Metab 2010;36:312–8.

68. Kanaya AM, Wassel Fyr CL, de Rekeneire N, Shorr RI, Schwartz AV, Goodpaster BH, et al. Predicting the development of diabetes in older adults: the derivation and validation of a prediction rule. Diabetes Care 2005;28:404–8.

69. Schmidt MI, Duncan BB, Bang H, Pankow JS, Ballantyne CM, Golden SH, et al. Identifying individuals at high risk for diabetes: The Atherosclerosis Risk in Communities study. Diabetes Care 2005;28:2013–8.
70. Griffin SJ, Little PS, Hales CN, Kinmonth AL, Wareham NJ. Diabetes risk score: towards earlier detection of type 2 diabetes in general practice. Diabetes Metab Res Rev 2000;16:164–71.
71. Park PJ, Griffin SJ, Sargeant L, Wareham NJ. The performance of a risk score in predicting undiagnosed hyperglycemia. Diabetes Care 2002;25:984–8.
72. Glümer C, Carstensen B, Sandbaek A, Lauritzen T, Jørgensen T, Borch-Johnsen K; inter99 study. A Danish diabetes risk score for targeted screening. Diabetes Care 2004;27:727–33.

CHAPTER 3

Diagnosis of prediabetes and diabetes prevention

Martin Buysschaert[1] and Michael Bergman[2]

[1] Department of Endocrinology and Diabetology, Université Catholique de Louvain (UCL),
University Clinic Saint-Luc, Brussels, Belgium
[2] Division of Endocrinology, NYU School of Medicine, NYU Diabetes and Endocrine Associates,
New York, NY, USA

Introduction

Type 2 diabetes is a metabolic disorder in which glucose is underutilized and overproduced, leading to hyperglycemia which is the hallmark of the disease. Insulin resistance and/or inadequate insulin secretion account for the progressive development of this condition, also previously referred to as non-insulin-dependent diabetes mellitus or adult-onset diabetes [1,2]. The World Health Organization (WHO) estimates over 180 million people suffer from diabetes worldwide and this number is projected to more than double by 2030 [3]. Chronic hyperglycemia of diabetes is associated with long-term damage of various organs, especially the eyes, kidneys, nerves, heart, and blood vessels [4].

Before the onset or diagnosis of overt type 2 diabetes, individuals may have significant "dysglycemia" for years, characterized by plasma glucose levels that do not meet the criteria for diabetes but are higher than those considered normal [1,5]. Diagnosis of the "prediabetic state" is mandatory because numerous clinical studies have indicated that a substantial number of individuals with this disorder will later develop diabetes and that the condition is associated with an increased risk of chronic complications, in particular cardiovascular events [6–12].

As dysglycemia is a biochemical marker of the prediabetic state, scientific societies before 2010 recommended that a blood glucose measurement serves as the exclusive method for diagnosing this condition. The most widely accepted glucose criteria were based upon fasting plasma glucose (FPG) or 2-h plasma glucose levels during a 75-g oral glucose tolerance test (OGTT). However, criteria and glycemic cutoff values for diagnosing the prediabetic state have been revised several times in the past decades. The National Diabetes Data Group (NDDG) in 1979 introduced the concept of "glucose intolerance," defined as a metabolic (hyperglycemic) state intermediate between normal glucose homeostasis and diabetes [5]. These criteria were promulgated in 1980 by the WHO [13]. In 1997, an International Expert Committee (IEC) convened by the American Diabetes Association (ADA) and the International Diabetes Federation (IDF), introduced the clinical entity termed "prediabetes" which comprises two pathophysiologic disorders: impaired fasting glucose (IFG) and impaired glucose tolerance (IGT) [1].

This chapter provides an overview of (i) the historical definitions of the prediabetic state and (ii) the status of current diagnostic criteria of prediabetes on the basis of long-standing glucose criteria (FPG and/or OGTT) and, more recently, the HbA1c (glycated hemoglobin) level.

Historical synopsis

The NDDG established a set of criteria defining both diabetes and the prediabetic condition referred to as glucose intolerance [5]. The criteria for diabetes were essentially based on the distribution of glucose levels within the general population and on blood glucose concentrations that predicted the development of diabetic retinopathy [14]. Diabetes was defined by an FPG $\geq$140 mg/dL or a 2-h value after a 75-g oral glucose challenge of $\geq$200 mg/dL. Glucose intolerance was identified by the presence of an FPG level <140 mg/dL, a glucose value of 140–199 mg/dL 120 minutes after an OGTT, and at least one other glucose concentration $\geq$200 mg/dL at 30, 60, or 90 minutes (Table 3.1). These recommendations were endorsed by the WHO. However, the WHO stated that glucose intolerance could be defined by a single glucose level of 140–199 mg/dL 120 minutes after OGTT if the FPG was <140 mg/dL. The requirement for an additional glucose measurement (at 30, 60, or 90 minutes) was dropped, possibly to simplify the process and in view of the relationship between the 2-h glucose value during the OGTT and development of microvascular complications [13].

In 1997, the IEC (convened by ADA and IDF) re-examined the diagnostic criteria in light of new information available since the original

Table 3.1 Diagnostic criteria for diabetes and "dysglycemia."

		Diabetes	"Dysglycemia"	
NDDG (1979) [5] National Diabetes Data Group	Fasting glucose[a] Casual glucose	≥140 (7.8) "Unequivocally elevated"	<140 (7.8) –	[GI][d]
	Symptoms OGTT (120 min)	++ ≥200 (11.1)[b]	– 140–199 (7.8–11.0)	
WHO (1980, 2006, 2011) [13,18,25] World Health Organization	Fasting glucose	≥126 (7.0)	110–125 (6.1–6.9)	[IFG[d]]
	Casual glucose Symptoms OGTT (120 min)	≥200 (11.1) ++ ≥200 (11.1)	– – 140–199 (7.8–11.0)	[IGT[d]]
	HbA1c (%)	≥6.5		
Expert Committee (1997) [1][c] Expert Committee on the Diagnosis and Classification of Diabetes Mellitus	Fasting glucose Casual glucose	≥126 (7.0) ≥200 (11.1)	110–125 (6.1–6.9) –	[IFG[d]]
	Symptoms OGTT (120 min)	++ ≥200 (11.1)	– 140–199 (7.8–11.0)	[IGT[d]]
Expert Committee (2003) [16][c] Expert Committee on the Diagnosis and Classification of Diabetes Mellitus	Fasting glucose Casual glucose	≥126(7.0) ≥200 (11.1)	100–125 (5.6–6.9) –	[IFG[d]]
	Symptoms OGTT (120 min)	++ ≥200 (11.1)	– 140–199 (7.8–11.0)	[IGT[d]]
ADA (2010) [21][c] American Diabetes Association	Fasting glucose Casual glucose Symptoms OGTT (120 min)	≥126 (7.0) ≥200 (11.1) ++ ≥200 (11.1)	100–125 (5.6–6.9) – – 140–199 (7.8–11.0)	[IFG[d]] [IGT[d]]
	HbA1c (%)	≥6.5	5.7–6.4	[IFG/ IGT][d]

[a]Plasma glucose values are expressed in mg/dL (mmol/L).
[b]In addition, at another time (30, 60, 90 min), a second value ≥200 mg/dL (11.1 mmol/L) is required.
[c]Diagnosis must be confirmed by repeat testing (in the absence of unequivocal clinical hyperglycemia).
[d]GI, glucose intolerance; IFG, impaired fasting glucose; IGT, impaired glucose tolerance. Both IFG and/or IGT are referred to as "prediabetes."

NDDG report [1]. An objective was to make the FPG and the 2-h glucose value during the OGTT equivalent for establishing the diagnosis of diabetes; if one criterion was met, the other would likely to be met as well. The IEC retained the 2-h glucose level of ≥200 mg/dL as an adequate criterion but lowered the FPG to ≥126 mg/dL (instead of ≥140 mg/dL). To justify the lowering of FPG, the IEC linked the new level (≥126 mg/dL) with the development of diabetic retinopathy in Pima Indians, Egyptians, and in a selected cohort of the Third National Health and Nutrition Examination Survey (NHANES III) [1]. The new criteria also included a formal diagnosis of diabetes in the presence of symptoms associated with a casual plasma glucose ≥200 mg/dL.

As a consequence of these changes, diagnostic criteria for "glucose intolerance" were also adopted. The IEC defined two new intermediate states of abnormal glucose regulation between normal glucose homeostasis and diabetes. IFG was defined by a FPG level of 110–125 mg/dL and IGT by a 2-h plasma glucose level during an OGTT of 140–199 mg/dL. These conditions representing different pathophysiologic processes were referred to as "prediabetes" in the new classification. FPG was the preferred test for screening but an OGTT could be required when diabetes was still suspected despite a normal FPG level. The WHO subsequently adopted most of these IEC/ADA/IDF conclusions but stated that individuals with IFG should undergo an OGTT to definitively exclude IGT or diabetes [15].

The previous FPG range for IFG of 110–125 mg/dL was further lowered in 2003 to 100–125 mg/dL [16]. The rationale for this decision was based on data suggesting that individuals with an FPG level of 100–109 mg/dL were already at increased risk for developing type 2 diabetes as well as to make the prevalence of IFG similar to that of IGT. As expected, the change in this cut-point increased considerably the overall prevalence of IFG, approximately three- to fourfold. Some experts did not support the latter decision [17] and the WHO still defines IFG with the previous FPG range (110–125 mg/dL) [18]. At that time, diagnosis of prediabetes using HbA1c was not recommended in part due to a lack of assay standardization.

In 2009, after an extensive review of biologic and epidemiologic evidence, the IEC (including representatives of ADA, IDF, and the European Association for the Study of Diabetes) recommended that diabetes and prediabetes could also be diagnosed by measuring the HbA1c (which reflects average blood glucose concentrations for the previous 2–3 months) [19–22]. Most studies indicated that there was an increased risk for retinopathy when HbA1c levels approximated 6.5% (comparable to the risk for corresponding FPG and IGT) [23,24]. Consequently, diabetes could be diagnosed by an HbA1c level ≥6.5% while individuals with an HbA1c level of ≥5.7–6.4% would be considered as having prediabetes or were at "increased risk for diabetes." The IEC suggested that the range of HbA1c (≥6.0 to <6.5%) represented the highest risk for the development of diabetes and that individuals with HbA1c levels <6% were also of concern, especially in the presence of other risk factors [20]. The WHO concurs with the use of HbA1c (≥6.5%) for defining diabetes but not for diagnosing prediabetes [25].

Current definition, mechanisms, and consequences of prediabetes

Since 2010, the ADA clinical practice guidelines define prediabetes ("increased risk for diabetes") as either IFG (fasting plasma glucose of 100–125 mg/dL) or IGT (2-h glucose during OGTT of 140–199 mg/dL) (Table 3.2). The recommendations also state that an HbA1c level of 5.7–6.4% identifies individuals at high risk for diabetes and that the term prediabetes could be applied [21,26].

People with isolated IFG predominantly have hepatic insulin resistance and normal muscle sensitivity, whereas individuals with isolated IGT have normal to slightly reduced hepatic insulin sensitivity but moderate to severe muscle insulin resistance. Individuals with IFG and IGT have both

Table 3.2 Increased risk for diabetes (prediabetes).[a,b]

FPG 100–125 mg/dL (5.6–6.9 mmol/L)	→ IFG
FPG <100 mg/dL (5.6 mmol/L) 2-h PG during the 75-g OGTT: 140–199 mg/dL (7.8–11.0 mmol/L)	→ IGT
HbA1C: 5.7–6.4%	→ IFG/IGT

FPG, fasting plasma glucose; IFG, impaired fasting plasma glucose; IGT, impaired glucose tolerance; OGTT, oral glucose tolerance test;
[a]For all three tests, the American Diabetes Association states that the risk is continuous, extending below the lower limit of the range and becoming disproportionately greater at higher ends of the range.
[b]A positive test result should be repeated using the same test for confirmation.
Source: Adapted from the International Expert Committee [20] and American Diabetes Association [21,26].

hepatic and muscle resistance. Individuals with isolated IFG have a decrease in the first phase (0–10 minutes) insulin secretory response to intravenous insulin, a reduced early phase (first 30 minutes) insulin response to oral glucose but a normal late phase (60–120 minutes) response during OGTT. Those with IGT also have a defect in early phase insulin secretion in response to oral glucose but, in addition, they also have a severe defect in late phase insulin secretion. HbA1c captures global glycemic excursions during the previous 2–3 months without specifying whether abnormalities are a consequence of pre- and/or postprandial glucose levels [27].

Prediabetes should be viewed as a risk factor presaging: (i) the development of diabetes; and (ii) an increase in cardiovascular (and possibly microvascular) complications. Current estimates from observational studies suggest that 25–40% of individuals with prediabetes will develop diabetes over the subsequent 3–8 years [28]. The average risk is about 5–10% per year compared with approximately 0.7% per year in normoglycemic individuals [8]. The incidence is highest in subjects with combined IFG and IGT and similar in those with IFG or IGT. Moreover, longitudinal studies suggest that prediabetes is mainly associated with an increased risk for cardiovascular events, with IGT and HbA1c being stronger risk predictors than IFG [9,29–31].

Testing for prediabetes: Methodologic and epidemiologic considerations

The identification of prediabetes permits intensive management to delay progression to diabetes and to prevent the development of chronic complications. However, the published literature lacks consensus as to which screening procedure for prediabetes (FPG, OGTT, HbA1c) is the most appropriate.

FPG, OGTT, and HbA1c: From a methodologic view

FPG has been widely accepted as an excellent diagnostic criterion for prediabetes. Advantages of FPG measurements include its ease and inexpensiveness with universally available automated instruments. Similarly, OGTT has been used for many years as another "gold standard" for the diagnosis of prediabetes [32].

Nevertheless, blood glucose measurements (FPG/OGTT) are subject to limitations in terms of high intraindividual and interindividual biologic variation, pre-analytic conditions and analytic variability which affect accuracy of diagnosis. Moreover, OGTT (which is time consuming and more expensive) has poor reproducibility [32–34].

HbA1c was recently included as an alternative diagnostic test as assays are now highly standardized and their results uniformly applicable across populations [21]. HbA1c has clearly superior attributes when compared with blood glucose criteria. Subjects need not fast and samples can be obtained at any time. The assay has little intraindividual variation, low pre-analytic instability and analytic variability. Interindividual variability is somewhat greater because HbA1c values may not be constant among all individuals despite similar blood glucose concentrations. HbA1c levels are higher in African Americans and Mexican Americans than in white individuals across the *continuum* of glycemia [35,36]. Other caveats include shortened erythrocyte lifespan, acute blood loss, and/or transfusions which lower HbA1c values as well as iron deficiency anemia, hypertriglyceridemia, uremia, and/or chronic alcohol consumption which slightly increase the level. Interference of hemoglobin variants can occur but are not a concern when appropriate assays (e.g., high performance liquid chromatography) are used [32–34]. Thus, generally, HbA1c can be measured accurately in the vast majority of individuals [37].

FPG, OGTT, and HbA1c: From an epidemiologic view

For decades, the diagnosis of prediabetes has been based on the FPG and/or on the 2-h glucose value after OGTT. As an increase in postprandial glucose concentrations occurs generally before the rise in FPG, the 2-h value during OGTT has been universally considered as a very early marker of impaired glucose homeostasis and a reliable indicator of risk for developing diabetes. OGTT is also a better predictor of cardiovascular morbidity and mortality than FPG, evidenced in the DECODE Study [30] and more recently by Ning et al. [38] in subjects within the normoglycemic range. As far as HbA1c is concerned, in agreement with ADA recommendations, Bonora et al. [39] demonstrated that a "high normal" HbA1c was an independent risk factor for developing diabetes during a 15-year follow-up period. Hazard ratio was 12.50 (95% CI 5.51–28.34) for a baseline HbA1c level of 6.00–6.49% (reference range 5.00–5.49%). Heianza et al. [40] and Inoue et al. [41] also indicated that the predictive value of an HbA1c range (5.7–6.4%) was similar to that assessed by IFG. The alternative of HbA1c for diagnosing (pre)diabetes was also based on outcomes from clinical studies demonstrating a strong relationship between HbA1c concentrations and microvascular complications as well as an increased prevalence of retinopathy starting with HbA1c levels approximating 6.5% [20,22,24]. HbA1c has also been considered an excellent predictor of cardiovascular disease and death [9]. The multiple adjusted hazard ratios were 1.78 (95% CI 1.48–2.45) and 1.25 (95% CI 1.53–2.48) for HbA1c ranges 5.5–6% and 6.0–6.5%, respectively [9]. Recently, Paynter et al. [42] found that HbA1c levels improved significantly the predictive ability of cardiovascular risk compared with classification of diabetes as a risk equivalent.

Nevertheless, the strategy of using HbA1c for detecting prediabetes has been questioned [43]. Cowie et al. [44] observed a substantially lower prevalence of undiagnosed "high risk for diabetes" by using HbA1c (range 6.0–6.5%) than detected with the FPG and OGTT (3.4 vs. 29% [IFG–IGT combined]). Similarly, Olson et al. [45], when comparing the performance of HbA1c (ranges 6.0–6.4% and 5.7–6.4%) with the OGTT, concluded that HbA1c criteria were less sensitive for screening. The report of Mann et al. [28], based on the NHANES 1999–2006 data, indicated that the prevalence of prediabetes among US adults was 12.6% by the HbA1c criterion and 28.2% by FPG and that the sensitivity and specificity for HbA1c for diagnosing prediabetes were 27% and 93%, respectively. Zhou et al. [46] in China and Heianza et al. [40] in Japan extended these observations and confirmed that blood glucose performed better than HbA1c. Mohan et al. [47], in the context of racially discrepant results of HbA1c, suggested that the cut-point for diagnosing prediabetes could be different in non-western than in western populations with an optimal threshold of 5.6% in Asian Indians. Glucose criteria were also considered as more precise correlates of insulin resistance and secretion than HbA1c in the Insulin Resistance Atherosclerosis Study [48]. Performance characteristics of HbA1c for the diagnosis of overt diabetes have been similarly debated [45,49,50]. Alternatively, HbA1c measurements may also lead to the reclassification of a considerable number of subjects without IFG to having prediabetes [28]. Findings from Abdul-Ghani et al. [51] could indirectly account for the latter observation as they demonstrated that an increase in the 1-h post glucose load (in the presence of a normal 2-h value) was associated with an increase in the incidence of type 2 diabetes.

Where are we now?

The use of absolute blood glucose and/or HbA1c cutoff values, inevitably required for clinical classification purposes, resulted in the definition of a new pathophysiologic entity. However, prediabetes should be considered as a risk factor for diabetes and cardiovascular disease rather than as a clinical entity [20]. Identification of prediabetes permits early intervention and management in order to delay progression to diabetes and to prevent the development of chronic complications, in particular macroangiopathy. It should be noted, however, that the evolution to diabetes may follow a *continuum* and could occur at blood glucose and HbA1c values lower than those meeting current definitions. Shaw et al. [52], Tirosh et al. [53], and Nichols et al. [54] reported that the risk of diabetes was already increased with FPG levels within the currently accepted normal range. Thus, an FPG of 90–94 mg/dL conferred a 49% greater risk of developing diabetes when compared with a level of less than 85 mg/dL [54]. In this study, aside from fasting glucose levels, the risk for developing diabetes was further increased by higher body weight and triglyceride levels. Similarly, Brambilla et al. [55] found that the glucose range 91–99 mg/dL demonstrated a hazard ratio of 2.03 (95% CI 1.18–3.50) versus hazard ratio of 1.42 (0.42–4.74) for the glucose range 83–90 mg/dL.

Analogously, there is substantial evidence that the curvilinear relationship between blood glucose levels and/or HbA1c with cardiovascular risk also extends below the prediabetes threshold, suggested by Hoogwerf et al. [56] and Selvin et al. [9]. In agreement with the ADA recommendations and noted by Bergman [57] and Buysschaert and Bergman [58], these "normoglycemic" patients may already be at risk, depending on the presence of other factors [47,48]. Tabak et al. [59] found a deviation from the linear trajectory in fasting and post-load glucose levels and insulin sensitivity 3–6 years prior to diagnosis. A "personalized" glucose profile has been proposed which may predict the gradual glycemic deterioration in a given individual who may then be encouraged to undertake early intervention [60]. Individuals demonstrating deteriorating glucose metabolism on a personalized level may not, however, be abnormal when a population-based standard is applied. Further studies are needed in order to better understand the clinical consequences of the "glycemic *continuum* theory."

Screening for prediabetes includes three methods of testing. HbA1c, in view of numerous clinical advantages, may be appealing to many primary care providers as the preferred method for screening. However, when used alone, the HbA1c may reclassify a large cohort of patients previously considered to have prediabetes to normal glycemic status and those without IFG to having prediabetes [28]. The impact of these observations remains unclear. The lower sensitivity of HbA1c at a designated cut-point may therefore offset its greater practicality [21]. Bonora and Tuomilehto [61] suggested that using both FPG and HbA1c as a reasonable option. Misra and Garg [62] and Heienza et al. [40] emphasized that the use of FBG and HbA1c together would also identify many more subjects at risk for diabetes and cardiovascular disease. Thus, if both tests results are above the diagnostic threshold, prediabetes would be confirmed. If the results are discordant, the test whose results are above the diagnostic cut-point could be repeated and the diagnosis would made on the basis of the confirmed test. Further studies on the pros and cons of using HbA1c versus glucose assays should continue until a more evidence-based consensus can be reached.

In conclusion, as the transition from a prediabetic state to overt type 2 diabetes clearly has clinical consequences, there are good reasons to identify precise categories of "increased risk" on the basis of current recommendations of the ADA. This would initiate, if needed, preventive strategies with their potential long-term benefits. This approach will continue to evolve and be refined with the availability of additional data from clinical and epidemiologic research.

References

1. Expert Committee on the Diagnosis and Classification of Diabetes Mellitus. Report of the Expert Committee on the Diagnosis and Classification of Diabetes Mellitus. Diabetes Care 1997;20:1183–97.
2. Ferrannini E, Nannipieri M, Williams K, Gonzales C, Haffner SM, Stern MP. Mode of onset of type 2 diabetes from normal or impaired glucose tolerance. Diabetes 2004;53:160–5.
3. Wild S, Roglic G, Green A, Sicree R, King H. Global prevalence of diabetes: estimates for the year 2000 and projections for 2030. Diabetes Care 2004;27:1047–53.
4. Buysschaert M. Diabétologie Clinique, 4th edn. Louvain-La-Neuve, Paris: De Boeck, 2011: pp.125–63.
5. National Diabetes Data Group. Classification and diagnosis of diabetes mellitus and other categories of glucose intolerance. Diabetes 1979;28:1039–57.
6. Diabetes Prevention Program Research Group. Reduction in the incidence of type 2 diabetes with lifestyle intervention or metformin. N Engl J Med 2002;346:393–403.
7. De Vegt F, Dekker JM, Jager A, Hienkens E, Kostense PJ, Stehouwer CD, et al. Relation of impaired fasting and postload glucose with incident type 2 diabetes in a Dutch population: the Hoorn Study. JAMA 2001;285:2109–13.
8. Aroda VR, Ratner R. Approach to the patient with prediabetes. J Clin Endocrinol Metab 2008;93(9):3259–65.
9. Selvin E, Steffes MW, Zhu H, Matsushita K, Wagenknecht L, Pankow J, et al. Glycated hemoglobin, diabetes and cardiovascular risk in nondiabetic adults. N Engl J Med 2010;362:800–11.

10. Diabetes Prevention Program Research Group. The prevalence of retinopathy in impaired glucose tolerance and recent-onset diabetes in the Diabetes Prevention Program. Diabet Med 2007;24:137–44.

11. Sumner CJ, Sheth S, Griffin JW, Cornblath DR, Polydefkis M. The spectrum of neuropathy in diabetes and impaired glucose tolerance. Neurology 2003;60:108–11.

12. Plantinga LC, Crews DC, Coresh J, Miller ER, Saran R, Yee J, et al. Prevalence of chronic kidney disease in US adults with undiagnosed diabetes or prediabetes. Clin J Am Soc Nephrol 2010;5:673–82.

13. World Health Organization. Diabetes mellitus: report of a WHO Study group. (Technical Report Series no. 646). Geneva: World Health Organization. 1980.

14. Pettitt DJ, Knowler WC, Lisse JR, Bennett PH. Development of retinopathy and proteinuria in relation to plasma-glucose concentrations in Pima Indians. Lancet 1980;ii:1050–2.

15. Alberti KG, Zimmet PZ. Definition, diagnosis and classification of diabetes mellitus and its complications. Part 1: diagnosis and classification of diabetes mellitus provisional report of a WHO consultation. Diabet Med 1998;15(7):539–53.

16. Expert Committee on the Diagnosis and Classification of Diabetes Mellitus. Follow-up report on the diagnosis of diabetes mellitus. Diabetes Care 2003;26:3160–7.

17. Davidson MB, Landsman PB, Alexander CM. Lowering the criterion for impaired fasting glucose will not provide clinical benefit. Diabetes Care 2003;26:3329–30.

18. World Health Organization. Definition and diagnosis of diabetes mellitus and intermediate hyperglycemia. Report of a WHO/IDF consultation. WHO/IDF 2006.

19. Saudek CD, Herman WH, Sacks DB, Bergenstal RM, Edelman D, Davidson MB. A new look at screening and diagnosing diabetes mellitus. J Clin Endocrinol Metab 2008;93(7):2447–53.

20. International Expert Committee. International Expert Committee Report on the role of the A1C assay in the diagnosis of diabetes. Diabetes Care 2009;32:1327–34.

21. American Diabetes Association. Standards of medical care in Diabetes, 2010. Diabetes Care 2010;33(Suppl.1):S11–S61.

22. Carson AP, Reynolds K, Fonseca VA, Muntner P. Comparison of A1c and fasting glucose criteria to diagnose diabetes among US adults. Diabetes Care 2010;33: 95–7.

23. Sabanayagam L, Liew G, Tai ES, Shankar A, Lim SC, Subramaniam T, Wong TY. Relationship between glycated haemoglobin and microvascular complications: is there a natural cut-off point for the diagnosis of diabetes? Diabetologia 2009;52: 1279–89.

24. Colagiuri S, Lee CMY, Wong TY, Balkau B, Shaw JE, Borch-Johnsen KB, for the DETECT-2 Collaboration Writing Group. Glycemic thresholds for diabetes-specific retinopathy. Diabetes Care 2011;34:145–50.

25. Report of a World Health Organization Consultation. Use of glycated haemoglobin (HbA1c) in the diagnosis of diabetes mellitus. Diabetes Res Clin Pract 2011;93: 299–309.

26. American Diabetes Association. Standards of medical care in diabetes, 2013. Diabetes Care 2013;36(Suppl.1):S1–S66.

27. Færch K, Borch-Johnsen K, Holst JJ, Vaag A. Pathophysiology and aetiology of impaired fasting glycemia and impaired glucose tolerance: does it matter for prevention and treatment of type 2 diabetes? Diabetologia 2009;52:1714–23.

28. Mann DM, Carson AP, Shimbo D, Fonseca V, Fox CS, Muntner P. Impact of A1c screening criterion on the diagnosis of pre-diabetes among US adults. Diabetes Care 2010;33:2190–5.
29. Khaw KT, Wareham N, Luben R, Bingham S, Oakes S, Welch A, et al. Glycated hemoglobin, diabetes, and mortality in men in Norfolk cohort of European Prospective Investigation of cancer and nutrition (EPIC-Norfolk). BMJ 2001;322:1–6.
30. Decode Study Group, on behalf of the European Diabetes Epidemiology Group. Glucose tolerance and cardiovascular mortality: comparison of fasting and 2-h diagnostic criteria. Arch Intern Med 2001;161:397–404.
31. Gerstein HC, Islam S, Anand S, Almahmeed W, Damasceno A, Dans A, et al. Dysglycemia and the risk of acute myocardial infarction in multiple ethnic groups: an analysis of 15,780 patients from the INTERHEART study. Diabetologia 2010;53:2509–17.
32. Sacks DB. A1c versus glucose testing: a comparison. Diabetes Care 2011;34:518–23.
33. Sacks DB, Arnold M, Bakris GL, Bruns DE, Horvath AR, Kirkman MS, et al. Position statement executive summary: guidelines and recommendations for laboratory analysis in the diagnosis and management of diabetes mellitus. Diabetes Care 2011;34:1419–23.
34. Sacks DB, Arnold M, Bakris GL, Bruns DE, Horvath AR, Kirkman MS, et al. Guidelines and recommendations for laboratory analysis in the diagnosis and management of diabetes mellitus. Diabetes Care 2011;34:e61–e99.
35. Ziemer DC, Kolm P, Weintraub WS, Vaccarino V, Rhee MK, Twombly JG, et al. Glucose-independent, Black–White differences in hemoglobin A1C levels. Ann Intern Med 2010;152:770–7.
36. Herman WH, Ma Y, Uwaifo G, Haffner S, Kahn SE, Horton ES, et al. for the Diabetes Prevention Program. Differences in A1c race and ethnicity among patients with impaired glucose tolerance in the diabetes prevention program. Diabetes Care 2007;30(10):2453–7.
37. Davidson MB. Diagnosing diabetes with glucose criteria: worshipping a false god. Diabetes Care 2011;34:524–6.
38. Ning F, Tuomilehto J, Pyörälä K, Onat A, Söderberg S, Qiao Q, for the DECODE Study Group. Cardiovascular disease mortality in Europeans in relation to fasting and 2-h plasma glucose levels within a normoglycemic range. Diabetes Care 2010;33:2211–6.
39. Bonora E, Kiechi S, Mayr A, Zoppini G, Targher G, Bonadonna RC, et al. High-normal HbA1c is a strong predictor of type 2 diabetes in the general population. Diabetes Care 2011;34:1038–40.
40. Heianza Y, Hara S, Arase Y, Saito K, Fujiwara K, Tsuji H, et al. HbA1c: 5.7–6.4% and impaired fasting plasma glucose for diagnosis of prediabetes and risk of progression to diabetes in Japan (TOPICS 3): a longitudinal cohort study. Lancet 2011;378:147–55.
41. Inoue K, Matsumoto M, Akimoto K. Fasting plasma glucose and HbA1c as risk factors for type 2 diabetes. Diabet Med 2008;25:1157–63.
42. Paynter NP, Mazer NA, Pradhan AD, Gaziano JM, Ridker PM, Cook NR. Cardiovascular risk prediction in diabetic men and women using hemoglobin A1c vs diabetes as a high-risk equivalent. Arch Intern Med 2011;171:1712–8.

43. Bloomgarden Z. A1C: recommendations, debates and questions. Diabetes Care 2009;32:141–7.
44. Cowie CC, Rust KF, Byrd-Holt DD, Gregg EW, Ford ES, Geiss LS, et al. Prevalence of diabetes and high risk for diabetes using A1C criteria in the U.S. population in 1988–2006. Diabetes Care 2010;33:562–8.
45. Olson DE, Rhee MK, Herrick K, Ziemer DC, Twombly JG, Phillips LS. Screening for diabetes and pre-diabetes with proposed A1c-based diagnostic criteria. Diabetes Care 2010;33:2184–9.
46. Zhou X, Pang Z, Gao W, Wang S, Zhang L, Ning F, et al. Performance of A1c and fasting capillary blood glucose test for screening newly diagnosed diabetes and pre-diabetes defined by an oral glucose tolerance test in Qingdao, China. Diabetes Care 2010;33:545–50.
47. Mohan V, Vijayachandrika V, Gokulakrishnan K, Anjana RM, Ganesan A, Weber MB, et al. A1c cut points to define various glucose intolerance groups in Asian Indians. Diabetes Care 2010;33:515–9.
48. Lorenzo C, Wagenknecht LE, Hanley AJG, Rewers MJ, Karter AJ, Haffner SM. A1c between 5.7 and 6.4% as a marker for identifying pre-diabetes, insulin sensitivity and secretion, and cardiovascular risk factors. Diabetes Care 2010;33(9):2104–9.
49. Lorenzo C, Haffner SM. Performance characteristics of the new definition of diabetes: the insulin resistance atherosclerosis study. Diabetes Care 2010;33:335–7.
50. Kramer CK, Araneta MRG, Barrett-Connor EB. A1c and diabetes diagnosis: the Rancho Bernardo Study. Diabetes Care 2010;33:101–3.
51. Abdul-Ghani MA, Stern MP, Lyssenko V, Tuomi T, Groop L, DeFronzo RA. Minimal contribution of fasting hyperglycemia to the incidence of type 2 diabetes in subjects with normal 2-h plasma glucose. Diabetes Care 2010;33:557–61.
52. Shaw JE, Zimmet PZ, Hodge AM, De Courten M, Dowse GK, Chitson P, et al. Impaired fasting glucose: how low should it go? Diabetes Care 2000;23:34–9.
53. Tirosh A, Shai I, Tekes-Manova D, Israeli E, Pereg D, Shochat T, et al. Israeli Diabetes Research Group.et al., for the Israeli Diabetes Research Group. Normal fasting plasma glucose levels and type 2 diabetes in young men. N Engl J Med 2005;353:1454–62.
54. Nichols GA, Hillier TA, Brown JB. Normal fasting plasma glucose and risk of type 2 diabetes diagnosis. Am J Med 2008;121:519–24.
55. Brambilla P, La Valle E, Falbo R, Limonta G, Signorini S, Cappellini F, et al. Normal fasting plasma glucose and risk of type 2 diabetes. Diabetes Care 2011;34:1372–4.
56. Hoogwerf BJ, Spreche DL, Pearce GL, Acevedo M, Frolkis JP, Foody JM, et al. Blood glucose concentrations ≤125 mg/dL and coronary heart disease risk. Am J Cardiol 2002;89:556–9.
57. Bergman M. Inadequacies of absolute threshold levels for diagnosing prediabetes. Diabetes Metab Res Rev 2010;26:3–6.
58. Buysschaert M, Bergman M. Definition of prediabetes. Med Clin North Am 2011;95(2):289–97.
59. Tabak AG, Jokela M, Akbaraly TN, Brunner EJ, Kivimaki M, Witte DR. Trajectories of glycaemia, insulin sensitivity and insulin secretion before diagnosis of type 2 diabetes: an analysis form the Whitehall II Study. Lancet 2009;373:2215–21.

60. Dankner R, Danoff A, Roth J. Editorial. Can 'personalized diagnostics' promote earlier intervention for dysglycaemia? Hypothesis ready for testing. Diabetes Metab Res Rev 2010;26:7–9.
61. Bonora E, Tuomilehto J. The pros and cons of diagnosing diabetes with A1c. Diabetes Care 2011;34(Suppl.2):S184–90.
62. Misra A, Garg S. HbA1c and blood glucose for the diagnosis of diabetes. Lancet 2011;378:104–6.

CHAPTER 4

What do we know about recruitment and retention in diabetes prevention programs? An Australian perspective

Philip Vita[1,5], Prasuna Reddy[2], Amy Timoshanko[3], Andrew Milat[4], Jane Shill[3], Alice Gibson[5], Greg Johnson[3] and Stephen Colagiuri[5]

[1] Sydney Diabetes Prevention Program, Sydney Local Health District, Sydney, NSW, Australia
[2] School of Medicine and Public Health, University of Newcastle, Callaghan, NSW, Australia
[3] Diabetes Australia – Victoria, Melbourne, VIC, Australia
[4] New South Wales Ministry of Health, North Sydney, NSW, Australia
[5] Boden Institute of Obesity, Nutrition, Exercise and Eating Disorders, University of Sydney, Sydney, NSW, Australia

Introduction

There is strong and consistent evidence from randomized controlled trials (RCTs) that type 2 diabetes can be prevented or delayed through lifestyle modification interventions that improve diet, increase physical activity, and achieve weight loss in people at high risk of developing the disease [1–7]. The Finnish [2] and United States (US) [7] studies achieved a 58% reduction, the Chinese study [1] a 35% reduction, the Indian study [8] a 29% reduction, and the Japanese (males only) study [3] a 68% reduction in type 2 diabetes incidence.

Moreover, the effects are sustained because the Finnish [9], US [10], and Chinese Da Qing studies [11] all demonstrated long-term diabetes risk reduction in those who were exposed to the interventions. The US study clearly demonstrated the cost effectiveness of this approach [12].

Additional quality controlled trials in Germany, Italy, and Iran have confirmed that lifestyle modification can prevent and/or delay the progression

Prevention of Diabetes, First Edition. Edited by Peter Schwarz and Prasuna Reddy.
© 2013 John Wiley & Sons, Ltd. Published 2013 by John Wiley & Sons, Ltd.

of type 2 diabetes [13–15]. Efficacy has been clearly established; however, most of these studies used intensive, individualized interventions that would be difficult to roll out in population-wide programs.

Recruitment in the landmark RCTs targeted people with abnormal glucose levels (either impaired fasting glucose (IFG) levels or impaired glucose tolerance (IGT)) requiring a range of blood tests including oral glucose tolerance tests (OGTT). Potential participants were selected based on age and selected risk factors such as family history. Recent community-based programs have used additional criteria based on standardized risk tools to screen and recruit participants [16,17].

Consequently, over the last 5 years there has been a plethora of translational research testing group-based programs and alternative screening and recruitment methods. A major focus of emerging translational research informing contemporary health policy is determining how best to utilize the limited resources for delivering lifestyle interventions to reach the greatest number of high-risk participants in the most efficient and cost-effective manner.

Researchers, policy makers, and practitioners often rely on evidence synthesis to inform the development of effective intervention programs. A number of systematic reviews and meta-analyses of lifestyle interventions in the prevention of type 2 diabetes have clearly established the "proof of concept" that diabetes can be prevented or delayed [5,18].

A quality systematic review and meta-analysis of 28 translation studies based on the US Diabetes Prevention Program demonstrated that at 12-months' follow-up, there was an average weight loss of 4% from baseline, which was similar regardless of whether the intervention was delivered by a health care professional or lay educator. Furthermore, with each additional lifestyle session attended, weight loss increased by 0.26 percentage points – supporting the dose–response relationship [19].

The challenge is now one of translation and scaling up of diabetes prevention programs into wider practice [20] and development and evaluation of pragmatic and sustainable strategies to identify and intervene in those at high risk in the community [21]. Inherent in this approach are the challenges in screening, recruiting, and retaining those who could benefit the most from these interventions [22–26]. In an environment of limited resources, intensive lifestyle interventions that capture a large number of the population who are unlikely to develop diabetes are not cost effective [27].

The objective of any parsimonious recruitment strategy is to screen and recruit people who are at high risk (without known or previously undiagnosed diabetes) and who would benefit from a lifestyle modification program and capture participants who will begin a lifestyle modification program and, equally importantly, complete it. Participants need to be made aware of their risk, be motivated to change, find a program that is convenient and appealing to them given their life circumstances, and be motivated to persist.

A wide range of recruitment strategies have been reported in the literature including direct mail to patients [28,29], workplace screening [17,30], facilitator led strategies [31], local level promotion and marketing [32], and participatory community-based strategies [33,34]. The development of epidemiologic-based risk tests has enabled the net to be cast wider and capture those who are at high risk and not just those with abnormal glucose levels [35,36].

Retention rates have not always been reported and comparisons between baseline characteristics of those who complete programs with those who do not are rarely reported. More importantly, there is a dearth of literature on predictors of program adherence.

We compared and contrasted two diabetes prevention programs in Australia: one a translational community-based program based in the primary health care setting, the Prevent Diabetes Live Life Well program (NSW, Australia), and the other a state-wide/regional roll out of a community-based program, Life! Taking Action on Diabetes (Victoria, Australia). Using both qualitative and quantitative methods we attempted to ascertain the critical success factors in screening and recruiting high-risk participants and also to determine what may encourage or hinder program completion. We describe each program in turn and then draw out the lessons learned in the discussion.

The Prevent Diabetes Live Life Well program

Description of the program

The Prevent Diabetes Live Life Well program (also known as the Sydney Diabetes Prevention Program) was funded by NSW Department of Health (state health authority) in 2008. The overall aim was to develop, implement, and evaluate an evidence-based lifestyle modification program to prevent or delay the onset of type 2 diabetes in high-risk English-speaking[1]

---

[1] The Prevent Diabetes Live Life Well program also targeted Arabic and Mandarin-speaking people, which is not reported here.

people aged 50–65 years [37]. Potential participants identified as being at high risk of developing type 2 diabetes (scoring ≥15 on the AUSDRISK questionnaire – a validated 10-item tool [36]) were screened and recruited by primary health care physicians (PHCPs) and were required to have previously undiagnosed diabetes excluded consistent with the national guidelines (Figure 4.1) [38]. PHCPs were recruited, orientated, and supported in running the program by the Divisions of General Practice (Divisions). Divisions are voluntary associations funded by the national government to assist primary health care settings to implement health promotion, early intervention/disease prevention, chronic disease management, medical education, and workforce support.

PHCPs were reimbursed a nominal fee for each referral. In total, 222 PHCPs were recruited and trained. There were two main screening and recruitment strategies trialed based on each PHCP's capacities and preferences: opportunistic and targeted.

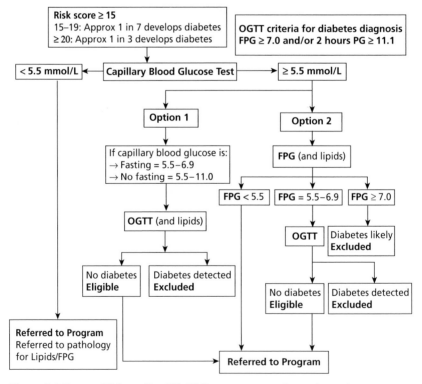

Figure 4.1 Prevent Diabetes Live Life Well program screening and recruitment process. FPG, fasting plasma glucose; OGTT, oral glucose tolerance test.

Opportunistic recruitment involved people being approached in the primary health care setting to complete the AUSDRISK tool by the PHCP or a practice staff member, or a member of the research team.

Targeted recruitment involved identifying people who were potentially eligible (within the age range, did not have an existing diagnosis of diabetes, or had certain risk factors – overweight or obese, high blood pressure, high cholesterol, family history) using the PHCP's clinical databases. They were either flagged on the daily appointment list or sent one of two types of letters to their home address: an invitation letter with a patient information sheet inviting them to come into the practice for screening, or an invitation letter with a brochure and the AUSDRISK tool to enable them to self-assess. Some primary health care settings followed up the letters with a phone call from a member of staff.

During the screening and recruitment period (September 2009 to June 2010) consistent feedback from the research staff running the program reported that the OGTT was a significant barrier to participants completing the eligibility requirements. Therefore, the screening process was modified to allow both fasting plasma glucose (FPG) and HbA1c [39] levels to be used to exclude diabetes instead of FPG and/or OGTT. This was taken up by some PCHPs and did appear to streamline the process and result in an increase in referrals.

In late 2009, the process was also modified to enable participants to be referred without having diabetes excluded by their PHCP. It was reported by lifestyle officers (LOs) that requiring pathology tests remained difficult for some participants who seemed to lose motivation and not complete the referral process. It was decided that as long as pathology results were received before participants attended groups or within 3 months of beginning the program they were included in the cohort (Figure 4.2).

Overall 70% of PHCPs referred at least one participant, and amongst this subsample the mean number of referrals was 14. The highest referring "champion" PHCP managed to refer 119 participants, demonstrating that with an appropriate system and support (motivated, personally interested, and delegating roles to each staff member, using a whole of primary care setting approach) it is feasible to screen and recruit participants through the primary health care setting.

Once eligible and recruited participants were contacted by the program providers and invited to attend an initial consultation the intervention was delivered by LOs who were employed through the Divisions. LOs were health professionals (psychologists, nurses, dietitians, diabetes educators, exercise physiologists) who undertook a minimum of 5 days of standardized

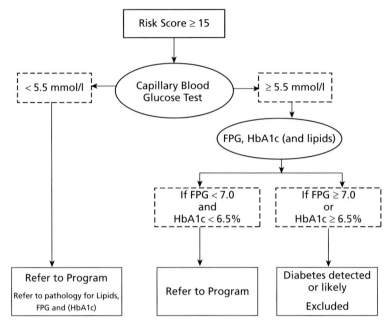

Figure 4.2 Prevent Diabetes Live Life Well program modified screening and recruitment process with HbA1c.

competency-based training. At the initial consultation participants were offered three 2-hour group lifestyle modification sessions (those who could not attend groups were offered an alternative individual telephone-based module), together with follow-up health coaching phone calls at 3, 6, and 9 months. Participants were recommended to seek ongoing support from their PHCP over the 12-month period and specifically asked to attend a 4-month PHCP review. Participants were also encouraged and supported to continue their lifestyle changes by being supplied with a list of "recommended" community-based physical activity and/or healthy eating services and facilities in their local area. At 12 months, participants attended a review session with their LO and PHCP for an end of program assessment. An outline of the program components are shown in Figure 4.3 [37].

Screening and recruitment outcomes
Over a 23-month period (September 2008 until June 2010), 4055 people consented to be screened, of whom 49% (n = 1983) were found to be at high risk (scored ≥15 on the AUDRISK). Of those at high risk, eligible, and

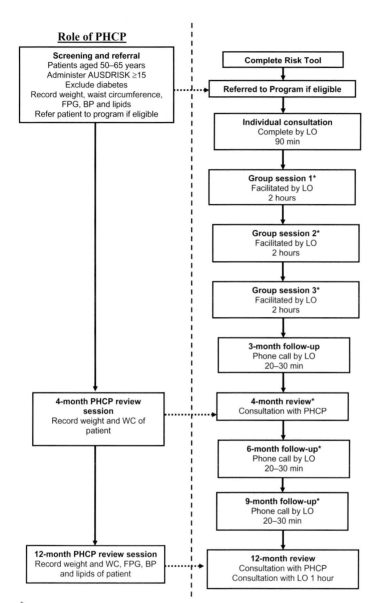

Figure 4.3 Prevent Diabetes Live Life Well program at a glance. BP, blood pressure; FPG, fasting plasma glucose; LO, lifestyle officer; PHCP, primary health care physician; WC, waist circumference.

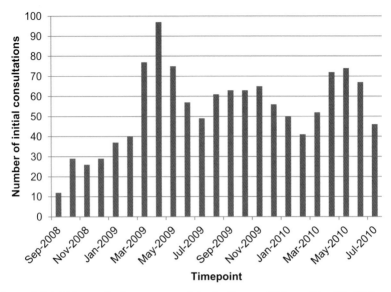

Figure 4.4 Initial consultations per month in the Prevent Diabetes Live Life Well program.

without undiagnosed diabetes (n = 1821), almost one-quarter (24%) declined to participate, leaving 1238 who began the program (mean age of 58 years; 63% female). The recruitment rates varied considerably over the recruitment period which probably reflected the staged approach to recruitment of the primary health care settings and PHCP, the increase in mail outs in early 2010, and various protocol amendments through the period (Figure 4.4).

A comparison with an age and region-matched representative population sample [40] found that the Prevent Diabetes Live Life Well program participants were more likely to be women, slightly more educated, had private health insurance, and were less likely to smoke or speak another language. Unfortunately, the reason why people (n = 435) chose to decline to take part in the program was not explored; however, as it was a free program it is unlikely that cost would have been a barrier.

Adherence and retention
In total, 880 participants had a 12-month review resulting in a completion rate of 71%. Twenty-two participants developed diabetes at the 12-month follow-up period (19 of whom attended a 12-month review) and a further 11 were excluded (being on weight loss and/or diabetes medication; having bariatric surgery; or not being able to determine their diabetes

status). Ultimately, there were 850 (69%) participants who completed ("completers") the 12-month program. Of the 19% (n = 234) who withdrew, the main factors given were personal (e.g., too busy with other commitments, family, or personal or social issues), rather than dissatisfaction with the program itself (e.g., program not helpful, cannot change their risk; did not like groups). The median time for withdrawal was 218 days (IQR 95–335). The overall loss to follow-up (withdrew or were unable to be contacted – "non-completers") was 29% (n = 350).

Comparisons of baseline characteristics of completers with non-completers found the later were significantly younger ($P < 0.01$), more likely to be receiving a pension ($P < 0.01$), less likely to be covered by private health insurance ($P < 0.001$), less likely to have a household income greater than \$100 000 ($P < 0.01$), and more likely to have a higher body mass index (BMI) ($P < 0.05$).

Regression analysis explored baseline predictors (age, sex, education, private health insurance, income, weight status, smoking status, alcohol consumption, self-efficacy, social support, mental health status) of program completion and time spent in the program. Completion was defined as attending the 12-month review and time spent in the program (total minutes) was based on participation at each contact point based on the following: initial consultation 90 minutes; group sessions, 120 minutes each; follow-up phone calls, 30 minutes each; 12-month review, 60 minutes. Therefore, the minimum time spent in the program was estimated at 90 minutes and the maximum time 600 minutes.

In terms of program adherence, the analysis revealed that participants who had private health insurance were 97% more likely to complete the program ($P < 0.0001$) and spent 24.6 minutes longer in the program ($P < 0.05$); for every year increase in age, the probability of completing the program went up by 5% ($P < 0.05$); participants who smoked spent 33.2 minutes less in the program ($P < 0.01$); participants who perceived social support from their PHCP to follow a healthy diet spent 30 minutes longer in the program ($P < 0.01$); and female participants spent 34.2 minutes longer in the program ($P < 0.01$).

Life! Taking Action on Diabetes program

Description of the program

Funded by the Victorian Department of Health, the Life! Taking Action on Diabetes program (Life! program) was launched in 2007 and is delivered by the non-government organization, Diabetes Australia – Victoria, the peak consumer body representing people affected by diabetes and those at risk in Australia. The aims of the Life! program are to:

- Raise community awareness of type 2 diabetes and prevention;
- Support targeted systematic risk assessment to identify those at high risk of developing type 2 diabetes;
- Deliver interventions that support the adoption of healthy and active lifestyles to reduce diabetes risk; and
- Contribute to earlier detection of type 2 diabetes in those who have undiagnosed type 2 diabetes, leading to better management and health outcomes.

The Life! program comprises three interventions: a group-based intervention (Life! course), Life! Telephone Health Coaching, and the Aboriginal Victorians Life! program. The main intervention and focus of this case study, the Life! course, is an evidence-based lifestyle behavior change program developed from several programs [41–43]. Centering on health psychology theories which focus on behavior change, including the self-regulation theory [44] and the Health Action Process Approach (HAPA) model [45], participants work towards adopting a healthier diet and active lifestyle to reduce their risk of developing type 2 diabetes.

The Life! course consists of six structured sessions of 1.5–2 hours' duration in groups of 6–18 participants. The "intensive phase" of the Life! course comprises five sessions conducted on a fortnightly basis. The sixth and final "maintenance" session is conducted 6 months following the intensive phase. Life! courses are delivered by trained facilitators (all qualified health care professionals) employed or contracted by public or private sector service providers, including community health services and medical centers. The Life! program has a payment system whereby providers are remunerated for each participant at three time points, dependent on attendance and completion of minimum participant data requirements for program evaluation.

Individuals at high risk of type 2 diabetes are identified using the Australian Type 2 Diabetes Risk Assessment tool (AUSDRISK) [36]. Individuals referred to the Life! program must have had diabetes excluded and have met one of the following sets of criteria: aged 50 years or older and have an AUSDRISK score of 12 or more; or aged 18 years and over and of Aboriginal or Torres Strait Islander decent with an AUSDRISK score of 12 or more; or have received a WorkHealth assessment (Victorian Government's worker health check program) [46]; or have a history of gestational diabetes mellitus (GDM) or ischemic heart disease (IHD).

To be eligible to participate in the Life! program it was initially required that all participants see their PHCP before commencement in order for diabetes to be excluded by pathology tests consistent with national guidelines [38]. This requirement proved a barrier to course commencement and potentially contributed towards participants losing motivation to commence a lifestyle modification program. This requirement was reviewed and participants are now able to participate in the Life! program as long as pathology tests are completed to exclude diabetes by the end of the intensive phase of the Life! course (session 5).

Recruitment

Critical to the successful implementation of a community-based prevention program is raising awareness in the community of both the problem and the preventative actions that can be taken. Three of the four key actions of the Life! program are based on increasing community awareness and identifying Victorians at risk of, or with currently undiagnosed, type 2 diabetes. All program promotion and communications have been based on key messages to increase and sustain awareness of: (i) the seriousness of diabetes; (ii) the opportunity to reduce risk with preventive actions; and (iii) and the existence of the Life! program, with the ultimate goal of facilitating program referrals. The Life! program had been accessed by over 22 000 Victorians at high risk of developing type 2 diabetes and this has been achieved by establishing multiple recruitment methods that provide a systematic and sustainable method of reaching and recruiting individuals at high risk of type 2 diabetes. Recruitment occurs via:

1. PHCPs and health professionals
2. Life! program service providers and facilitators
3. Direct engagement of the general public through Life! program social marketing campaigns
4. Engagement and recruitment in the workplace.

The current referral rate is over 11 000 referrals per year, with most being generated from facilitators/providers, PHCP/health professionals, and from self-referrals which are most likely a result of social marketing strategies (Figure 4.5).

PHCPs and health professionals

Engaging general practice and working closely with health professionals to identify high-risk individuals has been important in establishing a sustainable referral base. To assist in the engagement of PHCPs, a partnership was established with the local peak body representing general practitioners.

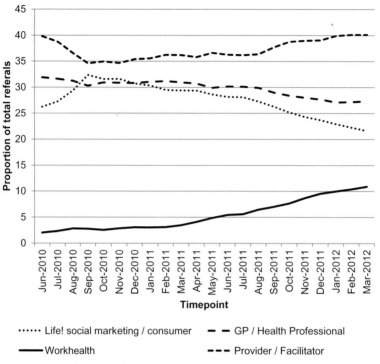

Figure 4.5 Proportion of total referrals from each Life! program referral method for the period June 2010 to March 2012.

To facilitate the targeted recruitment of high-risk individuals, a "case-finding" strategy was also implemented to provide a modest financial incentive to primary health care clinics for identifying and referring high-risk individuals to the Life! program. As seen in Figure 4.5, this initiative and engagement has resulted in approximately 30% of all program referrals.

Life! program providers and facilitators

Life! program service providers and facilitators are engaged in the Life! program not only as service providers, but also to recruit potential participants. Service providers have the potential to generate referrals into the Life! program by embedding promotion and delivery of Life! into internal systems within their organizations so that the Life! program effectively becomes part of routine service within an organization. Access to resources, start-up funding, and ongoing support has been provided to encourage promotion and recruitment activity in the local community, for example at local events and community gatherings.

Direct engagement of the general public through the Life! program social marketing campaign

The Life! social marketing strategy acted as an auxiliary to the other program engagement activities but was a standalone systematic application of marketing programs. Marketing for the Life! program has been comprehensive and incorporated mass media campaigns, social marketing, and targeted communication activities. Calls-to-action included 13RISK – a 24-hour telephone helpline, the Life! Program web site, and print publications which could be completed and returned to order a prevention kit. As of March 2012, there had been over 29 000 call-to-action responses and 407 908 AUSDRISK tools distributed to the public, Life! facilitators, and medical professionals.

Mass media campaigns and targeted communication activities have had a significant impact on the number of people contacting the Life! program, with spikes in call-to-action responses occurring during these activities. For example, Figure 4.6 shows a spike in referrals generated through the social marketing/self-referral method for the July–September 2010 quarter;

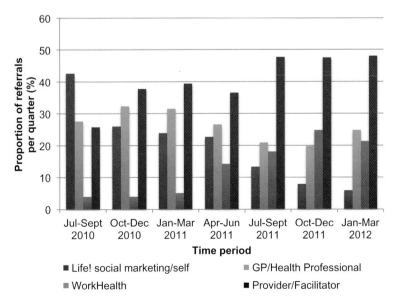

Figure 4.6 Proportion of referrals from each Life! program referral method each quarterly period from July 2010 to March 2012.

a television campaign was run in the months preceding this spike. The majority of people contacting the Life! program through the telephone helpline reported having heard about the program through advertising.

Social marketing research has been critical to establish an understanding of the target population and subsequently tailor marketing strategies to maximize engagement with and recruitment of the target population. Focus group testing indicated it was important to promote the Life! program as evidence-based, run by professionals, and tailored to the individual, as well as communicating practical information such as cost (free in most cases), time commitment, and that courses were available in the local area. An additional development to assist recruitment of participants has been the introduction of a central referral service. This service involves a number of follow-up telephone calls to an individual who has contacted the Life! program, providing a personalized point-of-contact between the individual and organization to assist the individual to maintain their motivation to commence the lifestyle modification course.

Workplaces

Workplace promotion to raise awareness about type 2 diabetes prevention and health amongst workers provides a significant opportunity to engage a large number of potential participants across a diverse range of the population, including people from low socioeconomic groups, varied education levels, and age groups. A tailored engagement program has been developed for workplaces which involves an employee dedicated to presenting sessions on type 2 diabetes and prevention. Furthermore, working in partnership with WorkHealth, the Life! program can be offered to workers at high risk of type 2 diabetes. As seen in Figure 4.5, the proportion of total referrals generated via WorkHealth is slowly increasing.

Retention and adherence

Participation in the Life! program is measured at three times points: attendance at Sessions 1, 5, and 6. An analysis was conducted on participant data from groups that had completed all sessions (n = 7314). Participants commencing Life! courses are on average 61.1 years old, female (66%), had completed secondary education (47%), had a low income level (53%), were non-smokers (91%), and were unemployed (47%). Analysis indicated good retention, with 76% (n = 5522) of individuals completing the intensive phase of the program. A regression analysis was conducted to explore factors that predicted completion of the intensive phase of the Life! program. Women and individuals with an education level higher than primary school were 15% and 43% more likely to complete the intensive phase, respectively. Interestingly, individuals who attended a Life! course conducted by a private provider were 30% more likely to complete the intensive phase. This may be because of payment for participant completion being a major source of business income for these providers, therefore increasing the importance of maximizing participant attendance. This finding suggests the need to investigate the strategies used by private providers to retain participants. Individuals from a culturally and linguistically diverse (CALD) background and individuals who smoked daily were 30% and 37% less likely to complete the intensive phase, respectively. Currently, individuals from CALD backgrounds attend mainstream courses with the assistance of a friend or family member for interpretation where required. Attrition may therefore occur as the course content is not culturally specific. The development of culturally appropriate strategies and service delivery options are ongoing.

A higher attrition rate is observed between sessions 5 and 6, with approximately 50% of participants dropping out after completion of the intensive phase. Feedback from Life! facilitators suggested that several factors contribute to the high attrition rate between these sessions. Results of a survey conducted in 2011 with over 100 facilitators indicated that many felt the 6-month gap between sessions 5 and 6 was too long, reporting it was difficult to keep participants engaged because they became demotivated and moved on to other priorities in their lives. Facilitators felt that positive group dynamics tended to contribute towards better attendance at the final session, and those individuals who had successfully achieved some behavior change and were enthusiastic and motivated to make further change were more likely to attend the final session. Similarly, focus groups (two groups, total n = 20) and in-depth interviews (n = 20) conducted with participants in 2011 who had completed the Life! course suggested participants also felt that the gap between sessions 5 and 6 was long, citing it was easy to forget the session or become demotivated to attend. However, participants did acknowledge that the 6-month period allowed them to make changes to their lifestyle and work towards the achievement of the Life! goals. These findings suggest the need to provide additional support between completion of the intensive phase and the final follow-up session, such as access to a telephone health coach or support via the internet. Some facilitators reported sending reminder letters or contacting participants by telephone before session 6. However, they reported varying levels of success in using this as a means of increasing participant retention.

Lessons learned

Screening for IGT in people at high risk of diabetes and intervening with lifestyle modification is a cost-effective health policy [47]. The challenges still remain in developing and implementing the most appropriate strategies to target those people at high risk who would benefit the most.

Key questions remain:
1. Where and how to recruit?
2. Who comes to lifestyle modification programs? Who misses out?
3. Who completes programs? Who drops out?

Where and how to recruit?

The findings from the Australian examples described here suggest that only using a single channel to screen and recruit – through the primary health care setting – results in limited impact. The Life! experience has demonstrated that having a population health focus with sustained social marketing and using multiple channels resulted in multiplying effects which increased referral rates. Program providers and facilitators who promoted the program were the most successful and this could have been in part because of their financial incentives. It was also encouraging that a growing proportion of referrals were from workplace strategies. In a large study in Greece it was found that recruiting in workplaces was more successful than in primary care [17]. The primary health care setting has been widely used with mixed results [34,48]. Future efforts to engage hard to reach segments of the population, including those who are medically underserved, will require tailored community-led strategies using lay people [49,50].

A whole community approach to encourage screening and recruitment using health promotion and education has been successful in Finland (Fin-2D2) [16,51]. Another population health example is in the Qingdao province in China where every household (1.94 million) received an educational booklet that contained a diabetes risk score with the aim of capturing high-risk individuals and channeling them into lifestyle counseling programs [52]. Social marketing is also pivotal in trying to reach those who are socioeconomically disadvantaged, as demonstrated in the New You New Life Program in the UK [53].

Who comes to programs?

We found that, consistent with other studies, even though men are at higher risk than women, it is women who are more likely to engage in diabetes prevention programs [19,54], and particularly those in which the main program components are delivered in face-to-face groups. Those recruited through the primary health care setting were more likely to be female, older, better educated, have higher incomes, not speak another language at home, and be less likely to smoke. Whereas those recruited through additional channels in the Life! program still captured more women than men, it appeared to recruit those who had lower socioeconomic status.

Demonstrated success in targeting and recruiting disadvantaged populations is emerging. For example, a diabetes prevention program in East Harlem, New York, using a targeted community-based approach, recruited 99 participants, of whom 58% had an education level less than high school; 70% were unemployed; 49% were uninsured; and 62% had a household income level of less than $15000 [34].

Screening and recruitment for diabetes prevention programs remains a complex process because of the requirement to exclude previously undiagnosed diabetes. The use of HbA1c to exclude diabetes does appear to streamline the process. Facilitating and supporting potential participants through the process shows great promise. Notwithstanding, diabetes prevention screening and recruitment needs to be more flexible, be delivered through a range of channels, and be supported by social marketing and information technology.

Who stays in programs?

The issue of adherence and retention is much more vexed. Dropout rates reported in the literature vary considerably [54]. The authors' experiences have shown that those who were older and female where more likely to complete programs, whereas those who were smokers were less likely. This could either be because participants change on their own, find the program is not what they expected, lose motivation, or have life circumstances that make it difficult for them to complete the program (other priorities in their lives). Having the support of a PHCP and/or family and friends increases adherence as did regular contact with program providers. For example, the Life! program found high attrition rates between group sessions 5 and 6 which were 6 months apart.

While the majority of studies report baseline characteristics of participants, further research is needed to differentiate the characteristics of completers from non-completers of interventions or programs. It is also important to review programs to determine factors that increase retention rates. Currently, financial incentives to participants and the use of lay health workers are showing promise.

Financial incentives and rewards to participants have been trialed in several ways [7,55,56]. For example, in a low socioeconomic status Latino community in Lawrence, Massachusetts, participants were given a cash incentive of $25 each for the baseline and 6-month visits, and $50 for completing the 12-month study [55]. This resulted in a retention rate of 93%. In one of four sites of the Montana Cardiovascular Disease and Diabetes Prevention Program participants were required to pay $50 at program entry and were then given $25 upon completion of the 16-week session and another $25 once they completed the 6-month follow-up session [56]. The overall completion rate of the 16-week intervention sessions across all four sites was 83% with no breakdown of each site. The high retention rates reported in these studies may be attributable to the financial incentives.

The use of lay community health workers has also been credited with high retention rates. The Group Lifestyle Balance study based on the original US Diabetes Prevention Program utilized lay health coaches, who were members of the study community, to implement the program [32]. The study had a retention rate of 77% which was attributed to the use of lay health coaches who "fostered a comfortable and familiar atmosphere for participants" [32, p.687].

Conclusions

There is emerging evidence that a population health or community-wide approach with a comprehensive social marketing strategy, telephone support, in a range of settings, particularly with program provider led strategies, holds great promise in capturing people at high risk of diabetes. Most programs continue be under-represented with males, the medically underserved, and those who are socially disadvantaged. However, the Life! program recruited those who had lower socioeconomic status. Adherence and retention remains a challenge. There is a need to investigate sustained multi-setting population health approaches targeting high-risk participants who are less likely to engage with and complete programs.

Acknowledgments

We would like to thank Dr. Jimmy Louie, University of Sydney, for assisting in the analysis of data.

Prevent Diabetes Live Life Well program

The program was funded by NSW Ministry of Health as part of the Australian Better Health Initiative with in-kind support provided by the Sydney Local Health District and the Australian Diabetes Council.

Chief investigators

Professor Stephen Colagiuri, University of Sydney

Professor Adrian Bauman, University of Sydney

Co-investigators/partners

Professor Maria Fiatarone Singh, University of Sydney

Professor Ian Caterson, University of Sydney

Associate Professor Marion Haas, University of Technology Sydney

Professor Chris Rissel, University of Sydney

Ms. Mandy Williams, South Western Sydney and Sydney Local Health Districts

Mr. Andrew Milat, NSW Ministry of Health

Dr. Warwick Ruscoe, Southern Highlands Division of General Practice

Dr. Michael Moore, Central Sydney GP Network

Mr. Rene Pennock, Macarthur Division of General Practice

Ms. Lilian Jackson, Australian Diabetes Council

Program staff

Magnolia Cardona-Morrell, Daniel Davies, Scott Dickinson, Louise Farrell, Alice Gibson, Melissa Gwizd, Jacky Hony, Sophia Lin, Kellie Nallaiah, Emma Sainsbury, and Philip Vita.

The Prevent Diabetes Live Life Well program would not have been possible without the perseverance and hard work of the primary health care physicians, lifestyle officers, and the program coordinators at the Central Sydney General Practice Network, Southern Highlands Division of General Practice, and the Macarthur Division of General Practice, respectively.

Most importantly, we would like to thank the participants who chose to be in the program and so generously provided their information.

Ethics approval to conduct the Prevent Diabetes Live Life Well program was granted by the Research Ethics Review Committee of the Sydney South West Area Health Service–Eastern Zone (ID number X08-0053).

Life! Program

The program was funded by the Department of Health, Victorian State Government.

The Life! Taking Action on Diabetes program would like to acknowledge the commitment of Life! program providers and facilitators in delivering Life! courses within the community.

References

1. Xiao-Ren P, Guang-Wei L, Ying-Hua H, Ji-Xing W. Effects of diet and exercise in preventing NIDDM in people with impaired glucose tolerance: the Da Qing IGT and diabetes study. Diabetes Care 1997;20(4):537–44.
2. Tuomilehto J, Lindstrom J, Eriksson JG, Valle TT. Prevention of type 2 diabetes mellitus by changes in lifestyle among subjects with impaired glucose tolerance. N Engl J Med 2001;344(18):1343–50.
3. Kosaka K, Noda M, Kuzuya T. Prevention of type 2 diabetes by lifestyle intervention: a Japanese trial in IGT males. Diabetes Res Clin Pract 2005;67(2):152–62.
4. Hussain A, Claussen B, Ramachandran A, Williams R. Prevention of type 2 diabetes: a review. Diabetes Res Clin Pract 2007;76(3):317–26.
5. Gillies CL, Abrams KR, Lambert PC, Cooper NJ, Sutton AJ, Hsu RT, et al. Pharmacological and lifestyle interventions to prevent or delay type 2 diabetes in people with impaired glucose tolerance: systematic review and meta-analysis. BMJ 2007; 334(7588):299–308.
6. Blackwell CS, Foster KA, Isom S, Katula JA, Vitolins MZ, Rosenberger EL, et al. Healthy living partnerships to prevent diabetes: recruitment and baseline characteristics. Contemp Clin Trials 2010;32(1):40–9.
7. Knowler WC, Barrett-Connor E, Fowler SE, Hamman RF, Lachin JM, Walker E, et al. Reduction in the incidence of type 2 diabetes with lifestyle intervention or metformin. N Engl J Med 2002;346(6):393–403.
8. Ramachandran A, Snehalatha C, Mary S, Mukesh B, Bhaskar AD, Vijay V. The Indian Diabetes Prevention Programme shows that lifestyle modification and metformin prevent type 2 diabetes in Asian Indian subjects with impaired glucose tolerance (IDPP-1). Diabetologia 2006;49(2):289–97.
9. Lindstrom J, Ilanne-Parikka P, Peltonen M, Aunola S, Eriksson JG, Hemio K, et al. Sustained reduction in the incidence of type 2 diabetes by lifestyle intervention: follow-up of the Finnish Diabetes Prevention Study. Lancet 2006;368(9548):1673–9.
10. Knowler WC, Fowler SE, Hamman RF, Christophi CA, Hoffman HJ, Brenneman AT, et al. 10-year follow-up of diabetes incidence and weight loss in the Diabetes Prevention Program Outcomes Study. Lancet 2009;374(9702):1677–86.
11. Li G, Zhang P, Wang J, Gregg EW, Yang W, Gong Q, et al. The long-term effect of lifestyle interventions to prevent diabetes in the China Da Qing Diabetes Prevention Study: a 20-year follow-up study. Lancet 2008;371(9626):1783–9.
12. Knowler WC, Barrett-Connor E, Fowler SE, Hamman RF, Lachin JM, Walker E, et al. Within-trial cost-effectiveness of lifestyle intervention or metformin for the primary prevention of type 2 diabetes. Diabetes Care 2003;26(9):2518–23.
13. Kulzer B, Hermanns N, Gorges D, Schwarz P, Haak T. Prevention of Diabetes Self-Management Program (PREDIAS): effects on weight, metabolic risk factors, and behavioral outcomes. Diabetes Care 2009;32(7):1143–6.

14. Azizi F, Rahmani M, Emami H, Mirmiran P, Hajipour R, Madjid M, et al. Cardiovascular risk factors in an Iranian urban population: Tehran Lipid and Glucose Study (Phase 1). Soz Praventivmed 2002;47(6):408–26.

15. Bo S, Ciccone G, Baldi C, Benini L, Dusio F, Forastiere G, et al. Effectiveness of a lifestyle intervention on metabolic syndrome: a randomized controlled trial. J Gen Intern Med 2007;22(12):1695–703.

16. Saaristo T, Moilanen L, Korpi-Hyovalti E, Vanhala M, Saltevo J, Niskanen L, et al. Lifestyle intervention for prevention of type 2 diabetes in primary health care. Diabetes Care 2010;33(10):2146–51.

17. Makrilakis K, Liatis S, Grammatikou S, Perrea D, Katsilambros N. Implementation and effectiveness of the first community lifestyle intervention programme to prevent type 2 diabetes in Greece: The DE-PLAN Study. Diabet Med 2010;27:459–65.

18. Yamaoka K, Tango T. Efficacy of lifestyle education to prevent type 2 diabetes: a meta-analysis of randomized controlled trials. Diabetes Care 2005;28(11): 2780–6.

19. Ali MK, Echouffo-Tcheugui J, Williamson DF. How effective were lifestyle interventions in real-world settings that were modeled on the Diabetes Prevention Program? Health Affairs 2012;31(1):67–75.

20. Milat AJ, King L, Bauman AE, Redman S. The concept of scalability: increasing the scale and potential adoption of health promotion interventions into policy and practice. Health Promot Int 2012; 12.

21. Simmons RK, Echouffo-Tcheugui JB, Griffin SJ. Screening for type 2 diabetes: an update of the evidence. Diabetes Obes Metab 2010;12(10):838–44.

22. Ruge T, Nystrom L, Lindahl B, Hallmans G, Norberg M, Weinehall L, et al. Recruiting high-risk individuals to a diabetes prevention program. Diabetes Care 2007; 30(7):e61.

23. Zhang P, Engelgau MM, Valdez R, Benjamin SM, Cadwell B, Venkat Narayan KM. Costs of screening for pre-diabetes among US adults. Diabetes Care 2003;26(9):2536–42.

24. Colagiuri S, Hussain Z, Zimmet P, Cameron A, Shaw J. Screening for type 2 diabetes and impaired glucose metabolism. Diabetes Care 2004;27(2):367–71.

25. American Diabetes Association. Screening for type 2 diabetes. Diabetes Care 2004;27(Suppl 1):s11–4.

26. Goyder E, Wild S, Fischbacher C, Carlisle J, Peters J. Evaluating the impact of a national pilot screening programme for type 2 diabetes in deprived areas of England. Fam Pract 2008;25(5):370–5.

27. Waugh N, Scotland G, Gillet M, Brennan A, Goyder E, Williams R, et al. Screening for type 2 diabetes: literature review and economic modelling. Research Report. Health Technol Assess 2007;11(17):1–146.

28. Schwarz P, Lindstrom J, Kissimova-Scarbeck K, Szybinski Z, Barengo N, Peltonen M, et al. The European perspective of type 2 diabetes prevention: Diabetes in Europe – Prevention using Lifestyle, physical Activity and Nutrition intervention (DE-PLAN) Project Exp Clin Endocrinol Diabetes 2008;116:167–72.

29. Kramer MK, Kriska AM, Venditti EM, Miller RG, Brooks MM, Burke LE, et al. Translating the Diabetes Prevention Program: a comprehensive model for prevention training and program delivery. Am J Prevent Med 2009;37(6):505–11.

30. Aldana S, Barlow M, Smith R, Yanowitz F, Adams T, Loveday L, et al. The Diabetes Prevention Program: a worksite experience. AAOHN J 2005;53(11):499–507.

31. Ackermann RT, Finch EA, Brizendine E, Zhou H, Marrero DG. Translating the Diabetes Prevention Program into the community: The DEPLOY pilot study. Am J Prevent Med 2008;35(4):357–63.

32. Seidel MC, Powell RO, Zgibor JC, Siminerio LM, Piatt GA. Translating the Diabetes Prevention Program into an urban medically underserved community. Diabetes Care 2008;31(4):684–9.

33. Horowitz CR, Eckhardt S, Talavera S, Goytia C, Lorig K. Effectively translating diabetes prevention: a successful model in a historically underserved community. Transl Behav Med 2011;1(3):443–52.

34. Parikh P, Simon E, Fei K, Looker H, Goytia C, Horowitz CR. Results of a pilot diabetes prevention intervention in East Harlem, New York City: Project HEED. Am J Public Health 2010;100(S1):S232–9.

35. Lindstrom J, Tuomilehto J. The diabetes risk score: a practical tool to predict type 2 diabetes risk. Diabetes Care 2003;26(3):725–31.

36. Chen L, Magliano DJ, Balkau B, Colagiuri S, Zimmet PZ, Tonkin AM, et al. AUS-DRISK: an Australian type 2 diabetes risk assessment tool based on demographic, lifestyle and simple anthropometric measures. Med J Aust 2010;192(4):197–202.

37. Colagiuri S, Vita P, Cardona-Morrell M, Singh M, Farrell L, Milat A, et al. The Sydney Diabetes Prevention Program: a community-based translational study. BMC Public Health 2010;10(1):328–35.

38. Colagiuri S, Davies D, Girgis S, Colagiuri R. National evidence based guideline for the case detection and diagnosis for type 2 diabetes. Canberra: Australia: Diabetes Australia and the NHMRC, 2009.

39. World Health Organization. Report of a World Health Organization consultation: use of glycated haemoglobin (HbA1c) in the diagnosis of diabetes mellitus. Diabetes Res Clin Pract 2010;93:299–309.

40. Centre for Epidemiology and Research. 2009 Report on adult health from the New South Wales Population Health Survey: 2009. Sydney, NSW: NSW Department of Health, 2010.

41. Uusitupa M, Lindi V, Louheranta A, Salopuro T, Lindstrom J, Tuomilehto J. Long-term improvement in insulin sensitivity by changing lifestyles of people with impaired glucose tolerance. Diabetes 2003;52(10):2532–8.

42. Laatikainen T, Dunbar J, Chapman A, Kilkkinen A, Vartiainen E, Heistaro S, et al. Prevention of type 2 diabetes by lifestyle intervention in an Australian primary health care setting: Greater Green Triangle (GGT) Diabetes Prevention Project. BMC Public Health 2007;7(1):249–56.

43. Moore SM, Hardie EA, Hackworth NJ, Critchley CR, Kyrios M, Buzwell SA, et al. Can the onset of type 2 diabetes be delayed by a group-based lifestyle intervention? A randomised control trial. Psychol Health 2011;26(4):485–99.

44. Oettingen G, Honig G, Gollwitzer P. Effective self-regulation of goal attainment. Int J Educat Res 2007;33:705–32.

45. Schwarzer R, Fuch R. Changing risk behaviours and adopting health behaviours: the role of self-efficacy beliefs. In: Bandura A, editor. Self-efficacy in Changing Societies. New York: Cambridge University Press; 1995: pp. 259–88.

46. WorkSafe Victoria. About WorkHealth. 2010 [April 2012]; Available from: (accessed 19 March 2013).

47. Palmer AJ, Tucker DMD. Cost and clinical implications of diabetes prevention in an Australian setting: a long-term modeling analysis. Prim Care Diabetes 2012;6(2) 109–21.

48. Gilis-Januszewska A, Szybinski Z, Kissimova-Skarbek K, Piwonska-Solska B, Pach D, Topor-Madry R, et al. Prevention of type 2 diabetes by lifestyle intervention in primary health care setting in Poland: Diabetes in Europe Prevention using Lifestyle, physical Activity and Nutritional intervention (DE-PLAN) Project. Br J Diabetes Vasc Dis 2011;11(4):198–203.

49. Horowitz CR, Brenner BL, Lachapelle S, Amara DA, Arniella G. Effective recruitment of minority populations through community-led strategies. Am J Prevent Med 2009;37(6):S195–200.

50. Murray NJ, Abadi S, Blair A, Dunk M, Sampson MJ, on behalf of the Norfolk Diabetes Prevention Study Group. The importance of type 2 diabetes prevention: The Norfolk Diabetes Prevention Study. Br J Diabetes Vasc Dis 2011;11(6):308–13.

51. Saaristo T, Peltonen M, Keinänen-Kiukaanniemi S, Vanhala M, Saltevo J, Niskanen L, et al. National type 2 diabetes prevention programme in Finland: FIN-D2D. Int J Circumpolar Health 2007;66(2):101–12.

52. Qiao Q, Pang Z, Gao W, Wang S, Dong Y, Zhang L, et al. A large-scale diabetes prevention program in real-life settings in Qingdao of China (2006–2012). Prim Care Diabetes 2010;4(2):99–103.

53. Penn L, Lordon J, Lowry R, Smith W, Mathers JC, Walker M, et al. Translating research evidence to service provision for prevention of type 2 diabetes: development and early outcomes of the "New life, New you" intervention. Br J Diabetes Vasc Dis 2011;11(4):175–81.

54. Jackson L. Translating the Diabetes Prevention Program into practice. Diabetes Educ 2009;35(2):309–20.

55. Merriam P, Tellez T, Rosal M, Olendzki B, Ma Y, Pagoto S, et al. Methodology of a diabetes prevention translational research project utilizing a community–academic partnership for implementation in an underserved Latino community. BMC Med Res Methodol 2009;9(1):20–9.

56. Amundson HA, Butcher MK, Gohdes D, Hall TO, Harwell TS, Helgerson SD, et al. Translating the Diabetes Prevention Program into practice in the general community. Diabetes Educ 2009;35(2):209–23.

CHAPTER 5

Depression and diabetes prevention

Norbert Hermanns

Department of Clinical Psychology, University of Bamberg, Bamberg, Germany; Research Institute of Diabetes Academy Mergentheim (FIDAM), Bad Mergentheim, Germany

Introduction

Diabetes mellitus is one of the most frequent metabolic disorders worldwide, characterized by persistent hyperglycemia. Epidemiologic data suggest that diabetes is a major global health problem. The International Diabetes Federation (IDF) estimates that 366 million people worldwide had diabetes in 2011 and that this will rise to 552 million people by 2030 [1]. The prevalence of diabetes in adults (aged 20–79 years) was estimated to be 6.4% in 2010 and will increase to 7.7% by 2030 worldwide. The total number of adults affected by diabetes will rise from 285 million in 2010 to 439 million by 2030 [2], because of changing population demographics, such as aging and urbanization, and changes in diet and physical activity, in part mediated through an increase in the prevalence of obesity and other lifestyle factors.

Depression is one of the most common mental health problems, affecting 4–7% of the population at any one time [3]. Almost one in five people can expect to experience a depressive disorder at some point in their lifetime. Depression affects about 121 million people worldwide. In 2000, depression was the leading cause of disability and the fourth leading contributor to the global burden of disease. The World Health Organization (WHO) estimates depression to reach second in the ranking of disability-adjusted life-years (DALYs) calculated for all ages and genders by the year 2020.

Besides their frequency and character as modern diseases of civilization, diabetes as a frequent metabolic disorder and depression as a common

Prevention of Diabetes, First Edition. Edited by Peter Schwarz and Prasuna Reddy.
© 2013 John Wiley & Sons, Ltd. Published 2013 by John Wiley & Sons, Ltd.

mental disorder seem to be linked with each other. This chapter reviews empirical evidence of the inter-relationship between diabetes and depression and focuses on possible mechanisms linking them. Consequences for clinical care as well as for research are outlined.

Depression as a risk factor for diabetes

The hypothesis that depression is a risk factor for diabetes was suggested 300 years ago by the British physician, Thomas Willis, who considered that diabetes might be a consequence of prolonged sorrows [4]. In the middle of the twentieth century, diabetes mellitus was listed as a psycho-somatic disease by Franz Alexander (1951), who assumed that intraper-sonal conflicts predispose individuals to diabetes.

In more recent years these historical observations have been supported by growing empirical evidence. A meta-analysis by Knol et al. [5] analyzed the impact of depression on the incidence of diabetes longitudinally. In this meta-analysis, nine studies were included which measured depression status at baseline in people without diabetes. After a follow-up period, which differed considerably between 3 and 16 years, diabetes incidence was assessed by self-report or laboratory measures. If depression or elevated depressive symptoms were present at baseline, the risk for diabetes increased for 37% (pooled hazard ratio 1.37, 95% CI 1.14–1.63) (Figure 5.1). Thus, it seems that depression or elevated depressive symptoms are

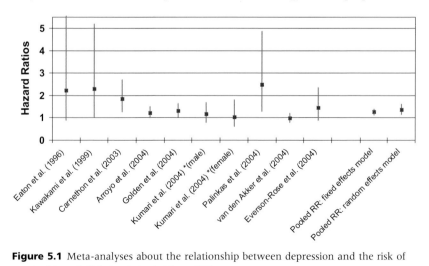

Figure 5.1 Meta-analyses about the relationship between depression and the risk of onset of type 2 diabetes (adapted from [5]).

a risk factor for non-diabetic people to go on to develop diabetes in the future. The authors stressed that mechanisms mediating elevated depressive symptoms or depression into the increased risk for diabetes are unknown [5].

Potential mechanisms linking diabetes and depression

Behavioral, inflammatory, and psychoendocrine mechanisms explaining the link between diabetes and antecedent depression are currently under research [6–9].

Behavioral mechanisms

Feelings such as loss of energy, withdrawal from daily activities, or sadness and low mood are key symptoms of depression. It seems common sense to assume that people affected by these symptoms are less likely to care for their health [10]. Regular physical activity and healthy eating to avoid obesity might be perceived as more difficult if depressive symptoms are present [10–12]. Lack of interest and reduced activity may predispose depressed people to not using the resources of the health care system for the detection and treatment of (metabolic) risk factors. Thus, it seems plausible that these behavioral factors could mediate depressive symptoms into an elevated diabetes risk in the long term.

Although the argument that an elevated risk of diabetes is mediated by lifestyle factors in depressed subjects is straightforward, new findings suggest that lifestyle factors are not the only explanation. Pan et al. [13] showed that depression (as assessed by clinical judgment or by questionnaire) increases the age-adjusted diabetes risk for 42% (hazard ratio 1.42, 95% CI 1.28–1.58). However, if lifestyle factors such as overweight, smoking, alcohol consumption, physical activity, eating behavior, and diet are taken into account in a multivariate model, the relative risk for diabetes is still significantly enhanced for 17% (hazard ratio 1.17, 95% CI 1.05–1.30). The comparison of the crude model with the full adjusted model shows that lifestyle factors can partially explain the elevated diabetes risk in depressed diabetic patients. However, the fact that the multivariate model is still significant after adjusting for these lifestyle factors shows that additional factors, not examined in this study, might have a role in mediating this elevated diabetes risk [13].

These results were confirmed independently by a longitudinal study by Golden et al. [14]. The crude hazard ratio showed a 12% rise (95% CI 1.03–1.21) in the diabetes risk per 5 unit increase on a depression scale. If lifestyle factors were adjusted for, the hazard ratio was reduced by 4 percentage points to 1.08 (95% CI 0.99–1.19), and the association was no longer statistically significant. In summary, it seems that lifestyle factors may partially explain an elevated diabetes risk in depressed people, but the risk elevation remains substantial even after adjusting for lifestyle factors, indicating that additional factors could be important.

Inflammatory mechanisms

Inflammatory processes as a possible link between diabetes and depression are currently receiving increased attention. The meta-analysis by Howren et al. [15] was able to demonstrate statistically significant associations between depression and inflammatory markers (CRP, C-reactive protein; IL-6, interleukin 6; IL-1, interleukin 1; and IL1-RA, interleukin 1 receptor antagonist). The strength of the associations between depression and these inflammatory markers were $d = 0.15–0.35$ if all studies were taken into account. If the meta-analysis was restricted to studies with clinical depressed subjects, the strength of associations increased remarkable to $d = 0.40$ (CRP), $d = 0.72$ (IL-6), $d = 0.41$ (IL-1), and $d = 0.31$ (IL1-RA). Thus, it seems that there is a dose–response relationship between severity of depression and inflammatory markers. More severe depression showed a stronger association to the abovementioned inflammatory markers than milder forms of depression.

Golden et al. [14] controlled the significantly elevated relative diabetes risk (hazard ratio 1.42, 95% CI 1.02–1.95) in depressed versus non-depressed people for inflammatory markers (CRP and IL-6). The adjustment for these inflammatory markers reduced the hazard ratio for diabetes to 1.35 (95% CI 0.98–1.86). After controlling for inflammation the association between depression and incident diabetes was no longer significant [14]. This indicates that these inflammation markers may have a substantial role in mediating the effects of depression into an elevated diabetes risk.

The population-based European Investigation into Cancer and Nutrition (EPIC) [16] study demonstrated that elevated CRP (hazard ratio 1.9, 95% CL 1.2–3.2) and IL-6 (hazard ratio 2.57, 95% CI 1.24–5.47) are significantly associated with an increased diabetes risk in the future.

The link between diabetes and inflammation is not only established epidemiologically, but also from interventional studies. Patients treated by anti-inflammatory drugs such as tumor necrosis factor (TNF) inhibitors or hydroxychloroquine for rheumatoid arthritis or psoriasis could significantly reduce their diabetes risk by 38% for TNF inhibitors (hazard ratio 0.62, 95% CI 0.42–0.82) and by 46% for hydroxychloroquine (hazard ratio 0.54, 95% CI 0.36–0.80), respectively [17]. An experimental treatment approach to type 2 diabetes with an anti-inflammatory therapy using an IL1-RA significantly reduced HbA1c 0.46 percentage points [18,19].

Chronic inflammatory processes are not only suspected to be associated with an elevated risk for diabetes and depression, but also with an increased likelihood for the development of atherosclerotic complications [20,21]. In summary, it seems that, besides lifestyle factors, inflammation could have a decisive role in the explanation of an increased diabetes risk.

Stress

An experimental study by Moberg et al. [22] demonstrated that acute mental stress was able to increase significantly the levels of contra-insulinary hormones such as cortisol, epinephrine, and growth hormone. Blood pressure was also elevated. In a glucose clamp study, the glucose levels increased to 8.0 mmol/L after mental stress compared with 6.8 mmol/L without mental stress.

Newly diagnosed diabetic patients reported more critical life events than people with normal glucose tolerance levels. These data suggest that chronic stress was present previous to diabetes manifestation [23]. In another study, more chronic stress such as working stress was associated with an increased incidence of type 2 diabetes. Low decision latitude and low sense of coherence significantly increased the diabetes risk (hazard ratios 2.2, 95% CI 1.0–4.8 and 3.7, 95% CI 1.2–5.7, respectively) [24]. A population-based study in western Finland examined the role of stress and critical life events in the pathogenesis of the metabolic syndrome. Pyykkönen et al. [25] demonstrated that stressful life events, particularly those related to finance and work, were associated with an increased risk of metabolic syndrome (hazard ratios 1.42, 95% CI 1.03–1.98; and 1.30, 95% CI 0.99–1.70, respectively).

In summary, it seems plausible that frequent activation of the hypothalamic–pituitary–adrenal (HPA) axis and sympathetic nervous system (SNS) by stress and insufficient coping strategies to deal with distress may increase the risk for diabetes [8,26].

Antidepressive medication

Several studies addressed the association of antidepressant medication use with the risk of developing diabetes. In the Diabetes Prevention Program, antidepressant use at baseline respectively continuous antidepressant use during the study significantly increased the risk for diabetes. The adjusted hazard ratios for diabetes while taking antidepressive medications were 2.25 (95% CI 1.38–3.66) and 2.60 (95% CI 1.37–4.94) in the placebo group and 3.48 (95% CI 1.93–6.28) and 3.39 (95% CI 1.61–7.13) in the lifestyle intervention group [27]. In the Health Professionals Follow-up Study (HPFS) and in the Nurses Health Studies (NHS I and II) a significantly increased diabetes risk in people using antidepressive medications was also observed. The effect still remained even after multivariate adjustment for known diabetes risk factors (pooled hazard ratio 1.30, 95% CI 1.14–1.49) [28]. In patients with more severe depressive disorders the intake of antidepressive drugs for more than 25 months in a moderate to high daily dosage was associated with an 84% increased risk of diabetes (hazard ratio 1.84, 95% CI 1.35–2.52) [29].

It seems that the intake of antidepressive medications is a risk factor for incident diabetes. More research is needed to determine whether the elevated diabetes risk is a consequence of a possible metabolic effect of antidepressive medications per se or if the severity of depression requiring antidepressive medication is responsible for the elevated diabetes risk. It should also be clarified if there are any specific substance effects on the diabetes risk.

Possible mechanisms mediating elevated depression symptoms or clinical depression into an elevated diabetes risk are associated with an activation of the innate immune system and a dysregulation of the HPA axis. The latter might result in an increase in inflammation markers as well as in a release of contra-insulinary hormones. Besides these inflammatory and neuroendocrine mechanisms the behavioral consequences of depression also promote an elevated diabetes risk. Further research is needed to clarify and explore these possible mediating mechanisms between depression and diabetes.

Depression has proven to be a risk factor for diabetes but behavioral mechanisms alone cannot explain the elevated incidence of diabetes in depressed people. Clearly, research is needed to clarify the abovementioned mechanisms linking depression and diabetes.

From a clinical perspective the current state of knowledge suggests that diabetes prevention programs should not only focus on changing lifestyle factors like eating behavior and physical exercise, but also elevated depressive symptoms or reduced well-being, or emotional barriers for lifestyle changes should be taken into account in modern diabetes prevention programs.

Emotional aspects in diabetes prevention

Non-pharmacologic diabetes prevention programs focus on the modification of lifestyle factors, because the evidence that type 2 diabetes can be avoided by a change in eating behavior and weight reduction as well as by increasing physical activity is overwhelming [30,31]. Since there is evidence that emotional distress can also have a role in the manifestation of diabetes, it seems reasonable to address not only lifestyle-related issues in intervention programs, but also emotional problems in living with an elevated diabetes risk.

Emotional problems typically associated with diabetes prevention include:
• Attitudes towards the diabetes and/or health risk;
• Barriers for changing eating and/or exercise behavior;
• Coping with problems in maintaining lifestyle changes in daily routine; and
• Daily difficulties that interfere with targeted lifestyle changes.

Diabetes prevention programs should also allow participants to share experiences in living with negative emotional feelings and reduced well-being with others.

In the following section some examples taken from the PREDIAS program [32,33], the tool box of the Diabetes Prevention Program [34], and the IMAGE toolkit [35] are presented on how to address emotional issues within modern diabetes prevention programs.

Attitudes towards diabetes and health risks

A major challenge with people at risk for type 2 diabetes is to motivate them to undertake preventive action. Some people have a lack of knowledge of diabetes risk factors; others may neglect these risks or have exaggerated worries about their health [36]. The consequences are either lack of motivation for lifestyle changes or emotions such as anxiety or sadness because of exaggerated worries about their health risks. Diabetes prevention programs can provide reliable information about health risks to allow people at risk to be able to assess their own health and diabetes risk. Therefore, diabetes prevention programs should provide easy to understand information on the way lifestyle factors influence health risks. This supports their motivation to learn more about their diabetes risks and to change their lifestyle patterns. Tools for assessing the individual risk profile can help people to reach a realistic appraisal of their own health risks [37]. This can motivate for lifestyle changes, but can also prevent exaggerated and unrealistic worries and anxiety about health status.

Barriers to lifestyle changes

Eating behavior is frequently determined by established eating patterns. Besides supplying energy, eating fulfills many other demands, determined by cultural factors as well as by habits [38]. Dining is a social event, providing the opportunity to meet people and to communicate in a congenial atmosphere. Eating times also structure the course of the day and determine family meetings and exchange. Changes to the frequency of and content of meals are sometimes perceived as a threat to these socially and culturally determined aspects and functions of eating. Therefore, barriers to changing eating behaviors and patterns are common.

Furthermore, eating is not only a response to feelings of hunger, but also sometimes a reaction to negative emotions such as feelings of stress, boredom, or sadness. Eating is sometimes received as a comfort for negative emotions. Changing eating habits could therefore also have a negative impact on well-being, if no better coping strategies for living with these negative emotions are offered.

These cultural, social, and regulatory functions for negative emotions related to eating might by an important barrier to achieving changes of eating patterns [39]. Diabetes prevention programs should therefore address these functions of eating. An individual analysis of the emotional aspects of eating can contribute to finding better coping strategies for living with negative emotions. Being aware of the social and cultural dimension of eating can assist in finding solutions for a reduced caloric intake, while maintaining the positive cultural and social aspects of eating. Analysis of the psychologic dimension of eating behavior will assist in selecting appropriate and realistic strategies for changing eating habits [40,41].

Becoming more physically active is frequently perceived as a major challenge in people with an elevated diabetes risk [38]. Negative experiences with physical exercise or a negative self-image can be major barriers to an increase in daily exercise [42]. Exploring attitudes to and previous experiences with physical exercise can help to select appropriate daily exercise levels. The exchange of views about physical exercise within a group of people sharing an elevated diabetes risk might help to modify barriers to exercise.

Maintaining lifestyle changes in daily routine

Many people with an elevated diabetes risk have previously tried to lose weight and to exercise more [43]. After a successful initial modification of lifestyle, many people find it difficult to maintain these behavior changes. A relapse into old eating and non-exercising patterns are very common. Feelings of frustration and disappointment about unsuccessful attempts are also very common. These previous negative experiences can be major barriers to a new attempt to make behavior changes towards a healthier lifestyle.

Diabetes prevention strategies should incorporate strategies for maintenance of the adopted lifestyle with regard to eating and physical exercise [44]. Such strategies usually consist of the establishment of a monitoring procedure for weight and physical exercise. The second component is to set up a plan of what to do if relapses into old lifestyle patterns occur. Planned interventions in these cases such as keeping an eating diary are helpful maintenance strategies. Such a record can help to reidentify risk situations with regard to eating and physical exercise, and to plan appropriate actions to avoid or modify such situations.

Another focus of maintenance strategies is assisting participants of diabetes prevention programs to develop realistic expectations about the difficulties of adopting a healthy lifestyle in the long term [45]. Many participants' expectations are overoptimistic and therefore unrealistic, and so the risk of failure is high. Alternative realistic expectations could take into account the possibility of a relapse into the "old lifestyle" and to regard this as expected rather than a proof of failure. The question should not be *if* a relapse into old habits of eating and physical activities occurs, but *how* to cope with these relapses successfully [39].

Other obstacles to healthy lifestyle changes

Many people who are at risk for type 2 diabetes have to establish and maintain a healthy lifestyle while coping with other difficulties. They may have occupational demands preventing regular physical exercise or establishing a new healthy diet. They may have family requirements such as caring for children, grandchildren, or parents. Frequent temptations at family occasions or offerings of food and drink can cause difficulties. Withdrawal from social activities or not fulfilling occupational expectations is often not an option.

Interventions assisting people to harmonize a healthy lifestyle with fulfilling social and occupational expectations are essential [46,47]. Group interventions have been found to be helpful. The exchange of experiences with other group members who have also difficulties in harmonizing social demands with a new healthy lifestyle can help people at risk to reflect on how to address these issues. Adopting successful strategies from other group members on how to establish and maintain a healthy lifestyle while fulfilling social roles in family and occupational settings is another benefit from group interventions. Providing self-assertiveness techniques on how to deal with tempting offers, while keeping on track with lifestyle goals without offending significant others or withdrawing from social contexts can be helpful. Problem-solving strategies on how to cope with daily difficulties that have the potential to affect healthy living should therefore be also be dealt with in diabetes prevention programs.

Negative emotional feelings and reduced well-being

Negative feelings and reduced well-being can be a side effect of lifestyle modification programs, because the negative effects of changing the individual's lifestyle are usually experienced immediately, while positive consequences, like reduction of risk for diabetes and cardiovascular disease, will only be rewarded in the future. Diabetes prevention programs should therefore give space for expressing negative emotions associated with lifestyle changes. In group interventions, participants can learn how other members experience emotional consequences of lifestyle changes. There might be different attitudes and cognitions about personal experiences. There is also the potential that people at risk for diabetes can adopt more functional ways of thinking about their lifestyle changes, which usually results in less negative feelings [42,48].

Besides being able to moderate group discussion about negative emotions, prevention program managers should be able to identify people with more severe mental health problems, who should be referred to a mental health specialist.

Effects of diabetes prevention programs on emotional well-being

PREDIAS is a group program for diabetes prevention that addresses lifestyle changes like weight reduction and increase of physical exercises and also the abovementioned psychologic aspects of life modification. The PREDIAS program consists of 12 lessons. The content of the program has been described elsewhere [32,33]. The impact of the PREDIAS program on psychologic well-being, depression, and anxiety symptoms was evaluated at the 12-month follow-up assessment [49,50]. The effects sizes (Cohen's d) were $d = 0.33$ for well-being, $d = 0.28$ for depressive symptoms, and $d = 0.49$ for anxiety symptoms (Figure 5.2). The impact on anxiety was significant greater in the PREDIAS group than in the control group. The effect sizes all represent a medium to large effect on well-being.

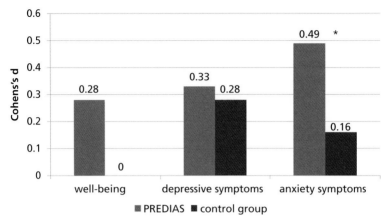

Figure 5.2 Effect size of a psychologic oriented diabetes prevention program (PREDIAS) on psychologic outcomes (adapted from [49,50]).

These results indicate that lifestyle changes are not necessarily associated with an increase in negative emotions. Addressing psychologic aspects in diabetes prevention programs was associated with positive effects on psychologic outcomes.

In summary, the PREDIAS study shows that psychologically sensitive diabetes prevention also results in an improvement in psychologic outcomes. Given that depression seems to be a risk factor for type 2 diabetes, it is encouraging that addressing emotional aspects of diabetes prevention is feasible and will result in a reduction of negative emotions like depression and anxiety, and an increase in psychologic well-being.

References

1. International Diabetes Federation. IDF Diabetes Atlas, 5th edn. Available from: http://www.idf.org/diabetesatlas/5e/the-global-burden (accessed 3 March 2013).
2. Shaw JE, Sicree RA, Zimmet PZ. Global estimates of the prevalence of diabetes for 2010 and 2030. Diabetes Res Clin Pract 2010;87(1):4–14.
3. Wittchen HU, Muller N, Pfister H, Winter S, Schmidtkunz B. Affektive, somatoforme und Angststörungen in Deutschland: Erste Ergebnisse des bundesweiten Zusatzsurveys "Psychische Störungen" [Affective, somatoform and anxiety disorders in Germany: initial results of an additional federal survey of "psychiatric disorders"]. Gesundheitswesen 1999;61:S216–222.
4. Willis T. Pharmaceutice rationalis sive diabtriba de medicamentorum operantionibus in humano corpore. Oxford: 1675.

5. Knol MJ, Twisk JW, Beekman AT, Heine RJ, Snoek FJ, Pouwer F. Depression as a risk factor for the onset of type 2 diabetes mellitus: a meta-analysis. Diabetologia 2006;49(5):837–45.
6. Brown AD, Barton DA, Lambert GW. Cardiovascular abnormalities in patients with major depressive disorder: autonomic mechanisms and implications for treatment. CNS Drugs 2009;23(7):583–602.
7. de Hert M, Dekker JM, Wood D, Kahl KG, Holt RI, Moller HJ. Cardiovascular disease and diabetes in people with severe mental illness position statement from the European Psychiatric Association (EPA), supported by the European Association for the Study of Diabetes (EASD) and the European Society of Cardiology (ESC). Eur Psychiatry 2009;24(6):412–24.
8. McIntyre RS, Rasgon NL, Kemp DE, Nguyen HT, Law CW, Taylor VH, et al. Metabolic syndrome and major depressive disorder: co-occurrence and pathophysiologic overlap. Curr Diab Rep 2009;9(1):51–9.
9. Pickup JC. Inflammation and activated innate immunity in the pathogenesis of type 2 diabetes. Diabetes Care 2004;27(3):813–23.
10. Gonzalez JS, Peyrot M, McCarl LA, Collins EM, Serpa L, Mimiaga MJ, et al. Depression and diabetes treatment nonadherence: a meta-analysis. Diabetes Care 2008;31(12):2398–403.
11. Ciechanowski PS, Katon WJ, Russo JE. Depression and diabetes: impact of depressive symptoms on adherence, function, and costs. Arch Intern Med 2000;160(21):3278–85.
12. Katon W, Cantrell CR, Sokol MC, Chiao E, Gdovin JM. Impact of antidepressant drug adherence on comorbid medication use and resource utilization. Arch Intern Med 2005;165(21):2497–503.
13. Pan A, Lucas M, Sun Q, Van Dam RM, Franco OH, Manson JE, et al. Bidirectional association between depression and type 2 diabetes mellitus in women. Arch Intern Med 2010;170(21):1884–91.
14. Golden SH, Lazo M, Carnethon M, Bertoni AG, Schreiner PJ, Diez Roux AV, et al. Examining a bidirectional association between depressive symptoms and diabetes. JAMA 2008;299(23):2751–9.
15. Howren MB, Lamkin DM, Suls J. Associations of depression with C-reactive protein, IL-1, and IL-6: a meta-analysis. Psychosom Med 2009;71(2):171–86.
16. Spranger J, Kroke A, Mohlig M, Hoffmann K, Bergmann MM, Ristow M, et al. Inflammatory cytokines and the risk to develop type 2 diabetes: results of the prospective population-based European Prospective Investigation into Cancer and Nutrition (EPIC)-Potsdam Study. Diabetes 2003;52(3):812–7.
17. Solomon DH, Massarotti E, Garg R, Liu J, Canning C, Schneeweiss S. Association between disease-modifying antirheumatic drugs and diabetes risk in patients with rheumatoid arthritis and psoriasis. JAMA 2011;305(24):2525–31.
18. Larsen CM, Faulenbach M, Vaag A, Ehses JA, Donath MY, Mandrup-Poulsen T. Sustained effects of interleukin-1 receptor antagonist treatment in type 2 diabetes. Diabetes Care 2009;32(9):1663–8.
19. Larsen CM, Faulenbach M, Vaag A, Volund A, Ehses JA, Seifert B, et al. Interleukin-1-receptor antagonist in type 2 diabetes mellitus. N Engl J Med 2007;356(15):1517–26.
20. Shishehbor MH, Bhatt DL. Inflammation and atherosclerosis. Curr Atheroscler Rep 2004;6(2):131–9.

21. Ridker PM, Silvertown JD. Inflammation, C-reactive protein, and atherothrombosis. J Periodontol 2008;79(8 Suppl):1544–51.
22. Moberg E, Kollind M, Lins PE, Adamson U. Acute mental stress impairs insulin sensitivity in IDDM patients. Diabetologia 1994;37(3):247–51.
23. Mooy JM, de Vries H, Grootenhuis PA, Bouter LM, Heine RJ. Major stressful life events in relation to prevalence of undetected type 2 diabetes: the Hoorn Study. Diabetes Care 2000;23(2):197–201.
24. Agardh EE, Ahlbom A, Andersson T, Efendic S, Grill V, Hallqvist J, et al. Work stress and low sense of coherence is associated with type 2 diabetes in middle-aged Swedish women. Diabetes Care 2003;26(3):719–24.
25. Pyykkonen AJ, Raikkonen K, Tuomi T, Eriksson JG, Groop L, Isomaa B. Stressful life events and the metabolic syndrome: the prevalence, prediction and prevention of diabetes (PPP)-Botnia Study. Diabetes Care 2010;33(2):378–84.
26. Golden SH. A review of the evidence for a neuroendocrine link between stress, depression and diabetes mellitus. Curr Diabetes Rev 2007;3(4):252–9.
27. Rubin RR, Ma Y, Marrero DG, Peyrot M, Barrett-Connor EL, Kahn SE, et al. Elevated depression symptoms, antidepressant medicine use, and risk of developing diabetes during the diabetes prevention program. Diabetes Care 2008;31(3):420–6.
28. Pan A, Sun Q, Okereke OI, Rexrode KM, Rubin RR, Lucas M, et al. Use of antidepressant medication and risk of type 2 diabetes: results from three cohorts of US adults. Diabetologia 2012;55:63–72.
29. Andersohn F, Schade R, Suissa S, Garbe E. Long-term use of antidepressants for depressive disorders and the risk of diabetes mellitus. Am J Psychiatry 2009;166(5):591–8.
30. Gillies CL, Abrams KR, Lambert PC, Cooper NJ, Sutton AJ, Hsu RT, et al. Pharmacological and lifestyle interventions to prevent or delay type 2 diabetes in people with impaired glucose tolerance: systematic review and meta-analysis. BMJ 2007;334(7588):299.
31. Orozco LJ, Buchleitner AM, Gimenez-Perez G, Roque IF, Richter B, Mauricio D. Exercise or exercise and diet for preventing type 2 diabetes mellitus. Cochrane Database Syst Rev 2008;3:CD003054.
32. Hermanns N, Gorges D. Primäre Diabetesprävention – PRAEDIAS – ein neues Schulungs und Behandlungsprogramm. Diabetes Aktuell 2007;5(2):54–64.
33. Hermanns N, Gorges D. PREDIAS: A structured treatment and education programme for prevention of type 2 diabetes. 2011. Available from: http://www.image-project.eu/pdf/PRAEDIAS.pdf (accessed 3 March 2013).
34. Diabetes Prevention Program Research Group. The Diabetes Prevention Program (DPP): description of lifestyle intervention. Diabetes Care 2002;25(12):2165–71.
35. Lindstrom J, Neumann A, Sheppard KE, Gilis-Januszewska A, Greaves CJ, Handke U, et al. Take action to prevent diabetes: the IMAGE toolkit for the prevention of type 2 diabetes in Europe. Horm Metab Res 2010;42(Suppl.1):S37–55.
36. Drapkin R, Wing R, Shiffman S. Responses to hypothetical high risk situations: do they predict weight loss in a behavioral treatment program or the context of dietry lapses? Health Psychol 1995;14:427–34.
37. Kanfer FH, Hagerman S. A model of self-regulation. In: Halisch F, Kuhl J, editors. Motivation, Intention and Volition. Berlin: Springer; 1987: pp. 293–307.
38. Biddle SHJ, Fox KR. Motivation for physical activity and weight management. Int J Obes (Lond) 1998;22(Suppl. 2):S39–47.

39. Bryne SM. Psychological aspects of weight maintenance and relapse in obesity. J Psychosom Res 2002;53:1029–36.

40. Delahanty LM, Meigs JB, Hayden D, Williamson DA, Nathan DM. Psychological and behavioral correlates of baseline BMI in the diabetes prevention program (DPP). Diabetes Care 2002;25(11):1992–8.

41. Gorges D, Kulzer B, Hermanns N, Schwarz P, Haak T. Psychologische und verhaltensbezogene Prädiktoren einer erfolgreichen Gewichtsreduktion in der Prävention des Typ 2 Diabetes. Diabetol Stoffwech 2009;4(Suppl.1):255.

42. McAuley E, Courneya K. Adherence to exercise and physical activity as health promoting behaviors: attitudinal and self-efficacy influences. Appl Prevent Psychol 1993;2:65–77.

43. Brownell KD, Jeffery RW. Improving long-term weight loss: pushing the limits of treatment. Behav Ther 1987;18:353–74.

44. Jeffery RW, Bjornson-Benson WM, Rosenthal BS, Lindquist RA, Kurth CL, Johnson SL. Correlates of weight loss and its maintenance over two years of follow-up among middle-aged men. Prevent Med 1984;13:155–68.

45. McGuire MT, Wing R.R., Klem ML, Lang W, Hill JO. What predicts weight regain in a group of sucessful weight losers. J Consult Clin Psychol 1999;67:177–85.

46. Gormally J, Rardin D. Weight loss and maintenance and changes in diet and exercise for behavioral counseling and nutritin education. J Counsel Psychol 1981; 28:295–304.

47. Dubbert PM, Wilson GT. Goal setting and spouse involvement in the treatment of obesity. Behav Res Ther 1984;22:227–42.

48. Klem ML, Wing R.R., Lang W, McGuire MT, Hill JO. Does weight loss maintenance become easier over time? Obes Res 2000;8:438–44.

49. Kulzer B, Hermanns N, Gorges D, Schwarz P, Haak T. Prevention of diabetes self-management program (PREDIAS): effects on weight, metabolic risk factors, and behavioral outcomes. Diabetes Care 2009;32(7):1143–6.

50. Kulzer B, Hermanns N, Gorges D, Schwarz P, Haak T. Effect of a diabetes prevention programme (PREDIAS) on metabolic risk factors and quality of life: results of a randomised controlled trial. Diabetologia 2010;53(Suppl.1):S83.

CHAPTER 6

Diabetes prevention in a challenging environment

Abdul Basit and Musarrat Riaz
Baqai Institute of Diabetology and Endocrinology (BIDE), Karachi, Pakistan

Pakistan is a developing country with diverse economic, educational, and social patterns. It has a population of 161.66 million, of whom 68% live in rural areas. Challenges faced by Pakistan are multifactorial: 30% (42 million) of the population live below the poverty line; 45% (61 million) of the population have no access to safe drinking water; and 40% (54 million) of the population have no access to even basic health services. Nine million children under the age of 5 years are malnourished and 8 million children do not go to school. Pakistan's education indicators are the worst in South Asia [1].

The health facilities available for the people of Pakistan are very poor. There are 149 201 registered doctors, with 1206 population per doctor. There are 10 958 registered dentists and 76 244 nurses [2]. There has been little increase in public sector spending in the health sector for the last 40 years. Since 1970, public expenditure on health and health infrastructure represented 0.7–0.8% of GDP and 3.5% of total government expenditure. Pakistan spends less than 30% of the health budget on the development of health infrastructure while private expenditure forms the bulk (75%) of total expenditure on health [3].

The International Diabetes Federation (IDF) estimates that there are approximately 7.1 million people with diabetes in Pakistan, ranking it seventh worldwide, and with the highest number of adults with diabetes [4]. This number is predicted to increase to 13.8 million by the year 2030, making it fourth in this list. These predictions are based upon population-based studies conducted in urban and rural areas of the four provinces of Pakistan at different periods, which show a prevalence of diabetes ranging

Prevention of Diabetes, First Edition. Edited by Peter Schwarz and Prasuna Reddy.
© 2013 John Wiley & Sons, Ltd. Published 2013 by John Wiley & Sons, Ltd.

3.7–16.2% in men and 4.8–11.7% in women. Similarly, prevalence of impaired glucose tolerance (IGT) ranges 4.5–8.2% in men and 5.8–14.3% in women [5–8].

The rates of complications of diabetes in Pakistan are alarmingly high. The frequency of people with coronary artery disease (CAD) is 15.1%, peripheral vascular disease (PVD) 5.5%, and cerebrovascular disease 4.5% [9]. Similarly, an estimated 15.9% of the population are affected by retinopathy, 4% with foot ulcers, and 8.4% with raised creatinine ± end stage renal disease (ESRD) [9–11].

The economic burden of treating diabetic complications is an important consideration. The average per capita health expenditure for 1 year is £1.7 (Rs. 220.58). The average direct cost of treating a University of Texas grade 1 diabetic foot ulcer is £21 (Rs. 2886), which is more than 10 times the average health expenditure of an average Pakistani household [12]. This means that 400 000 people with foot ulcers in Pakistan (i.e., 0.22% of the population) needs double the total health budget.

According to the World Health Organization (WHO), projections for Pakistan over the next 10 years are that deaths from chronic diseases will increase by 27% and deaths from diabetes are expected to increase by 51%. In 2005 alone, Pakistan lost 1 billion dollars in national income from premature deaths and will further lose 31 billion dollars over the next 10 years if solutions are not implemented [13].

Reasons identified for the increasing risk of developing diabetes in South Asians are manifold and include increased incidence of abdominal obesity, insulin resistance, and metabolic syndrome compared with other populations [14,15]. South Asians have increased diabetes and CAD at lower body mass index (BMI) than Europeans. Hence, both the WHO and IDF have recommended different BMI cutoff points for Asians (i.e., BMI >23 kg/m^2 is defined as overweight and BMI >25 kg/m^2 is defined as obesity). Similarly, South Asians are likely to have more visceral fat at any BMI score than Europeans, which is associated with a higher degree of insulin resistance for the same BMI [16]. In an epidemiologic survey of urban Karachi, Pakistan, metabolic syndrome was studied in adults aged 25 years or above. A total of 840 subjects were screened from the population of 699 595 through random selection of 500 households. It was observed that 68% of women and 46% of men were obese according to the Asian cutoff for waist circumference [17]. Similarly, using the BMI criteria for Asians in another study carried out in Hub, 18% were found to be obese while 27% were overweight [18]. Prevalence of metabolic syndrome was found to be 18–46% [18].

The increase in the prevalence of type 2 diabetes is predominantly in middle-aged people, partly because of the rising prevalence of childhood obesity. The National Health Survey of Pakistan 1990–1994 revealed that 1% of country's population was obese (BMI >30 kg/m^2) and 5% were overweight (BMI >25 kg/m^2) in the 15–24 year age group [19]. A similar study in 8- to 10-year-old school children of urban Karachi showed 4.3% to be obese, and 9.8% were found to be overweight. This study also showed that a large proportion of school children had modifiable risk factors of diabetes such as physical inactivity, unhealthy dietary habits, and increased BMI [20–22]. Frequency of certain modifiable risk factors (e.g., overweight and physical inactivity) was observed to be higher among children with a positive family history of diabetes, children belonging to upper income groups, and those living in urban areas [22–25]. A positive impact of behavioral interventions has been noted in this high-risk group [25].

Malnourishment amongst pregnant mothers is also not uncommon. It exposes the offspring to intrauterine growth retardation (IUGR) and compromised metabolic potential [26]. Maternal mortality rate and low birth weight are two important indicators of maternal malnutrition and rates of both are high in Pakistan [27]. There is a lack of data at national level regarding the frequency of overweight or body fat percentage among children with low birth weight. However, a pilot study regarding the effects of maternal health on glucose homeostasis of offspring showed that incidence of low birth weight (<2.5 kg) in undernourished mothers was 11.1%, whereas in normally nourished groups it was 7.4%. Further, cord blood glucose was higher (94.6 ± 35.8 vs. 83.2 ± 38.1 mg/dL) and cord insulin concentration was lower (11.4 ± 11.5 vs. 12.5 ± 17.44 pmol/L) in newborn infants of undernourished mothers compared with normally nourished mothers [28]. This pilot study is to be followed by a longitudinal study in which expectant mothers from first trimester will be recruited and followed up till term and analyzed for nutritional status and its impact on cardiometabolic status in newborn babies.

A recent study was carried out in the rural area of Baluchistan to observe the temporal changes in the prevalence of diabetes, impaired fasting glucose, and its associated risk factors. This community-based survey of 1264 subjects aged 25 years and above was conducted in 2010 in 16 villages of southern Baluchistan. The temporal changes were assessed in comparison with a similar survey conducted 7 years previously. A twofold increase in the prevalence of diabetes (from 7.2% to 14.2%) was seen. Similarly, the prevalence of impaired fasting glucose also increased significantly (6.5% to 11.0%) (Figure 6.1) [29].

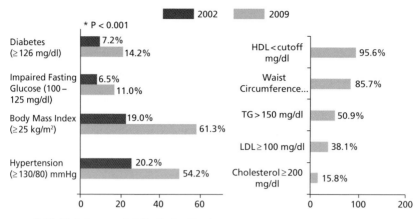

Figure 6.1 Temporal changes in the prevalence of diabetes in the rural area of Baluchistan, Pakistan (2002–2009) [29].

Studies have demonstrated that lifestyle modifications focused on losing weight, increasing physical activity, and improving diet could reduce the risk of progression to diabetes by nearly 60% [30,31]. In several randomized trials, drug therapy has also proven effective in the prevention of type 2 diabetes. A prospective primary prevention study has recently been completed in Pakistan [32]. The Diabetic Association of Pakistan (DAP) and Baqai Institute of Diabetology and Endocrinology (BIDE) has worked in collaboration with the University of Oslo (UIO). A high-risk group was identified on the basis of a predefined questionnaire for an oral glucose tolerance test (OGTT). These subjects were recruited from public awareness programs held at clinics and various organizations and institutes. The intervention program included a group with lifestyle modifications (LSM) that incorporated diet with exercise, a group on drug therapy (metformin) and a group on drug and lifestyle modification (Figure 6.2). A total of 47 incident cases of diabetes were diagnosed (overall incidence was 4 cases per 1000 person-months, with an incidence of 8.6 cases in the control group, 2.5 cases in the LSM group, and 2.3 cases in the LSM + drug groups). The study showed that lifestyle intervention had a major impact in preventing diabetes among IGT subjects in this region. Adding the drug did not improve results. The results of this preventive program will help in starting a large-scale public awareness program in the future.

Despite various challenges, the non-pharmacologic lifestyle approach to prevention of diabetes is highly effective. Diabetes prevention and control

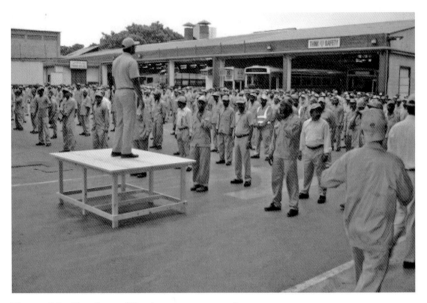

Figure 6.2 Lifestyle modification program at a factory.

are particularly relevant in countries like Pakistan because of increased inherent predisposition, young age of onset, and lack of capacity to treat the condition effectively at the primary health care level. Similarly, lack of equitable access to health care for the treatment of possible complications makes a strong case for investment in diabetes prevention and control. Prevention of type 2 diabetes requires a reliable system, not only to collect local data, but also to assess and monitor the situation in order to formulate guidelines for proper management. In Pakistan, lack of surveillance and diabetes research at national level are basic hindrances to developing programs to control the epidemic of type 2 diabetes.

A great challenge in primary prevention of diabetes is implementation of these trials in regional and national programs. Screening high-risk individuals with OGTT is costly and time consuming. Further, it is inconvenient and needs a physician to interpret results, making it impractical for mass screening programs. For this reason, various risk scores have been developed and validated in various populations, which have been shown to be effective in identifying people at risk of developing type 2 diabetes [30]. However, some of the Caucasian-derived risk scores have been found to be of low predictive value in South Asian populations, suggesting that risk scores may need to be developed that are relevant to the specific population [33,34]. Thus, a risk score RAPID (Risk Assessment of Pakistani Individuals for Diabetes), based on a self-assessment questionnaire, has been recently published and is expected to help to create a base for initiating mass public awareness programs in future. The questionnaire includes questions on age, family history of diabetes, and waist circumference [35]. These parameters are easy to understand and readily available for use to identify people at high risk of developing diabetes as well as identifying undiagnosed diabetes. In future, the use of simple cost-effective measures like mobile and internet technology for lifestyle modification will be utilized for massive awareness campaigns.

Primary prevention of diabetes has yet not received attention from the health department of the government of Pakistan; however, there are certain programs at governmental level that can be helpful (e.g., maternal and child health programs, girl nutrition program). In 1995, National Action Plans were made for control of diabetes [36] and in 2004 diabetes was recognized as one of the main chronic diseases needing national level strategies to control the rising epidemic of this disease [37].

Non-governmental organizations are also playing an important part in the prevention of type 2 diabetes by arranging continuous educational programs for health care providers as well as patients. Awareness campaigns for communities have contributed to primary prevention and control of diabetes in Pakistan. The Diabetic Association of Pakistan [36] has made a major contribution by serving as the WHO collaborating center for diabetes and conducted national diabetes surveys [5–8] in all provinces of Pakistan.

The recognition of diabetes and endocrinology as a separate sub-specialty by the College of Physicians and Surgeons, Pakistan (CPSP) is a major step forward in developing a faculty for secondary and tertiary care diabetes units. BIDE in Karachi is also contributing significantly by educating health care professionals. A 1-year Diploma in Diabetology for family physicians is regularly conducted by BIDE and 258 doctors in 12 batches have completed this course. Similarly, BIDE also offers a 1-year university-based Diploma in Diabetes Education and 83 educators have successfully completed this course. Peripheral Diabetes Centres (PDCs) have been established throughout Pakistan with the help of these diploma holders. These centers are actively engaged in various clinical research and educational activities in collaboration with BIDE, including primary prevention of diabetes. On the basis of its services, BIDE was awarded the status of IDF recognized center of diabetes education [38].

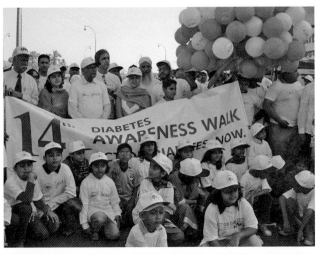

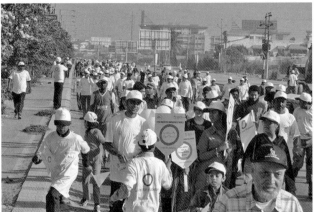

Figure 6.3 Diabetes Awareness walk.

The media has also started to have an important role in promoting the cause of primary prevention. Print and electronic media including FM radio and TV programs are now a regular feature being used efficiently to convey the message. Annual walks on World Diabetes Day are organized by government and non-governmental organizations, not only in major cities, but also in small cities, semi-urban, and rural areas (Figure 6.3).

Recently, the National Association for Diabetes Educators of Pakistan (NADEP) has been established with the aim of empowering people to prevent and control diabetes [39]. Continuous medical education programs, lectures, seminars, and symposia are organized regularly for family physicians, medical students, and other allied health care professionals. In addition to basic and advanced courses related to various aspects of diabetes prevention and management, public awareness programs and media campaigns are now a regular feature of primary prevention strategies. Special attention has been focused on children and school awareness programs are regularly conducted to increase the awareness of children regarding modifiable risk factors for the primary prevention of diabetes.

Development of the network, Active in Diabetes Prevention, has helped tremendously in a global view of experiences in various environments [40]. A book has been published on primary prevention by Schwarz et al. which has been very successful. The global diabetes survey has helped generate the intellectual input from health care professionals and colleagues interested in this important mission. World congresses on prevention of diabetes have given an impetus to the drive against this epidemic. IDF through Bridges has taken the initiative in its contribution towards primary prevention by announcing the D-Start program [41]. Pakistan has been selected as an implementation site for a primary prevention program along with Vietnam, the coordinating site being Finland. All these steps will help in creating an environment and mobilization of resources for promoting healthy lifestyles and prevention of type 2 diabetes in Pakistan.

References

1. Pakistan Statistical year book: 2005. Government of Pakistan, Statistics Division Federal Bureau of Statistics.
2. Pakistan economic survey 2011–2012, Government of Pakistan, Ministry of Finance, Islamabad. Available from: http://www.finance.gov.pk/survey/chapter_12/11-Health AndNutrition.pdf (accessed 25 March 2013).
3. Human Development in South Asia: The Health Challenge, 2004. Available from: http://www.mhhdc.org/reports/HDRSA%202004.pdf (accessed 4 March 2013).
4. International Diabetes Federation (IDF) Atlas, 4th edn. 2009.
5. Shera AS, Rafique G, Khwaja IA, Ara J, Baqai S, King H. Pakistan National Diabetes Survey: prevalence of glucose intolerance and associated factors in Shikarpur, Sindh Province. Diabet Med 1995;12:1116–21.
6. Shera AS, Rafique G, Khwaja IA, Baqai S, Khan IA, King H. Pakistan National Diabetes Survey prevalence of glucose intolerance and associated factors in North West at Frontier Province (NWFP) of Pakistan. J Pak Med Assoc 1999;49:206–11.
7. Shera AS, Rafique G, Khawaja IA, Baqai S, King H. Pakistan National Diabetes Survey: prevalence of glucose intolerance and associated factors in Baluchistan province. Diabetes Res Clin Pract 1999;44:49–8.

8. Shera AS, Basit A, Fawwad A, Hakeem R, Ahmedani MY, Hydrie MZ, et al. Pakistan National Diabetes Survey: prevalence of glucose intolerance and associated factors in the Punjab Province of Pakistan. Prim Care Diabetes 2010;4:79–83.

9. Basit A, Hydrie MZI, Hakeem R, Ahmedani MY, Masood Q. Frequency of chronic complications of type 2 diabetes. J Coll Physicians Surg Pak 2004;14:79–3.

10. Shera AS, Jawad F, Maqsood A, Jamal S, Azfar M, Ahmed U. Prevalence of chronic complications and association in type 2 diabetes. J Pak Med Assoc 2004;54:54–9.

11. International Diabetes Federation (IDF) Diabetes Atlas, 2nd edn. 2003.

12. Ali SM, Fareed A, Humail SM, Basit A, Ahmedani MY, Fawwad A, Miyan Z. The personal cost of diabetic foot disease in developing world: a study from Pakistan. J Diabet Med 2008;25:1231–3.

13. World Health Organization. Facing the facts: The impact of chronic disease in Pakistan. Available from: http://www.who.int/chp/chronic_disease_report/media/pakistan.pdf (accessed 4 March 2013).

14. Misra A, Wasir J, Vikram N. Waist circumference criteria for the diagnosis of abdominal obesity are not applicable uniformly to all populations and ethnic groups. Nutrition 2005;21:969–76.

15. Misra A. Insulin resistance syndrome (metabolic syndrome) and obesity in Asian Indians: evidence and implications. Nutrition 2004;20:482–91.

16. WHO Expert Consultation. Appropriate body-mass index for Asian populations and its implications for policy and intervention strategies. Lancet 2004;10;363(9403):157–63.

17. Hydrie MZI, Shera AS, Fawwad A, Basit A, Hussain A. Prevalence of metabolic syndrome in urban Pakistan (Karachi): comparison of newly proposed IDF and modified ATP III Criterions. Metab Syndr Relat Disord 2009;7:119–24.

18. Basit A, Samad Shera A. Prevalence of metabolic syndrome in Pakistan. Metab Syndr Relat Disord 2008;6(3):171–5.

19. National Health Survey of Pakistan 1990–1994: health profile of the people of Islamabad, Pakistan. PMRC; 1997: pp. 181.

20. Hydrie MZ, Basit A, Naeema B, et al. Diabetes risk factors in middle income Pakistani school children. Pak J Nutr 2004;3:43–9.

21. Basit A, Hakeem R, Hydrie MZI, Ahmedani MY, Masood Q. Relationship among fatness, blood lipids and insulin resistance in Pakistani children. J Health Popul Nutr 2005;23:34–43.

22. Misra A, Basit A, Vikram NK, et al. High prevalence of obesity and associated risk factors in urban children in India and Pakistan. Diabetes Res Clin Pract 2006; 71:101–2.

23. Hakeem R, Thomas J, Badruddin SH. Urbanisation and coronary heart disease risk factors in South Asian children. J Pak Med Assoc 2001;51:22–8.

24. Sheikh Rashid A, Jabbar A, Michels RP, DeVries JH. Metabolic risk factors, insulin-resistance and lifestyle in children of type 2 diabetes patients in Karachi, Pakistan. Diabetes Res Clin Pract 2008;80:399–404.

25. Badruddin SH, Molla A, Khursheed M, Vaz S. The impact of nutritional counselling on serum lipids, dietary and physical activity patterns of school children. J Pak Med Assoc 1993;43:235–7.

26. Corvalan C, Gregory CO, Ramirez-Zea M, Martorell R, Stein AD. Size at birth, infant, early and later childhood growth and adult body composition: a prospective study in a stunted population. Int J Epidemiol 2007;36:550–7.

27. Ministry of Health, Government of Pakistan. Nutritional Indicators. Ministry of Health, Government of Pakistan. 7-9-2010. Available from: www.health.gov.pk (accessed 4 March 2013).

28. Shaikh F, Basit A, Hakeem R, et al. Maternal health during pregnancy and cardio metabolic status of children at birth. Poster discussion in World Diabetes Congress held in Dubai, UAE, 4–8 December, 2011.

29. Basit A, Danish Alvi SF, Fawwad A, Ahmed K, Yakoob Ahmedani M, Hakeem R. Temporal changes in the prevalence of diabetes, impaired fasting glucose and its associated risk factors in the rural area of Baluchistan. Diabetes Res Clin Pract 2011;94:456–62.

30. Jaakko T, Jaana L, Johan GE, et al. Prevention of type 2 diabetes mellitus by changes in lifestyle among subjects with impaired glucose tolerance. N Engl J Med 2001; 344:1343–50.

31. Knowler WC, Barrett-Connor E, Fowler SE, Hamman RF, Lachin JM, Walker EA, et al. Reduction in the incidence of type 2 diabetes with lifestyle intervention or metformin. N Engl J Med 2002;346:393–403.

32. Hydrie MZI, Basit A, Shera AS, Hussain A. Effect of intervention in subjects with high risk of diabetes mellitus in Pakistan. J Nutr Metab 2012; Jul 19 [Epub ahead of print].

33. Mohan V, Sandeep S, Deepa M, Gokulakrishnan K, Datta M, Deepa R. A diabetes risk score helps identify metabolic syndrome and cardiovascular risk in Indians: the Chennai Urban Rural Epidemiology Study (CURES-38). Diabetes Obes Metab 2007;9:337–43.

34. Mohan V, Deepa R, Deepa M, Gokulakrishnan K, Datta M, Deepa R. A simplified Indian diabetes risk score for screening for undiagnosed diabetic subjects (CURES-24). J Assoc Physicians India 2005;53:759–63.

35. Riaz M, Basit A, Hydrie MZI, Shaheen F, Hussain A, Hakeem R, et al. Risk assessment of Pakistani individuals for diabetes (RAPID). Prim Care Diabetes 2012; 6:297–302.

36. Hakeem R, Fawwad A. Diabetes in Pakistan: epidemiology, determinants and prevention. J Diabetol 2010;3:4. Available from: http://www.journalofdiabetology.org/Pages/Releases/FullTexts/ThirdIssue/RA-1-JOD-10-039.aspx (accessed 25 March 2013).

37. Nishtar, S. National Action Plan for the prevention and control of non-communicable diseases and health promotion in Pakistan: cardiovascular diseases. World Health Organization, Ministry of Health, Government of Pakistan and Heart file. 2004. Available from: http://www.heartfile.org/pdf/NAPmain.pdf (accessed 4 March 2013).

38. International Diabetes Federation (IDF). IDF Centres of Education. Available from: http://www.idf.org/idf-centres-education (accessed 4 March 2013).

39. National Association of Diabetes Educators of Pakistan (NADEP). National Association of Diabetes Educators of Pakistan (NADEP). Available from: http://www.bideonline.com/nadep.aspx (accessed 4 March 2013).

40. Network Active in diabetes prevention. Available from: www.activeindiabetesprevention.com (accessed 4 March 2013).

41. Bridges: International Diabetes Federation. Available from: http://www.idf.org/bridges/d-start (accessed 4 March 2013).

CHAPTER 7

Global migration and prevention of diabetes

Bishwajit Bhowmik[1], Victoria Telle Hjellset[2] and Akhtar Hussain[1]

[1] Institute of Health and Society, Faculty of Medicine, University of Oslo, Oslo, Norway
[2] Institute of General Practice and Community Medicine, Department of Preventative Medicine and Epidemiology, University of Oslo and Norwegian University of Life Science, Oslo, Norway

Diabetes mellitus is a chronic metabolic disease characterized by elevated blood glucose levels resulting from the body's inability to produce insulin or depleted insulin action, or both.

There are two main forms of diabetes. Type 1 diabetes usually accounts for only a minority of the total burden of diabetes; it is the predominant form of the disease in younger age groups, mostly in high income countries, especially in the Nordic countries. However, evidence suggests that type 1 diabetes is increasing both in rich and poor countries.

Type 2 diabetes accounts for about 85–95% of all diabetes. Once considered a disease of affluence, type 2 diabetes is now a global health priority. It is one of the major contemporary causes of premature disability and death. In virtually every developed nation, diabetes ranks as one of the top two causes of blindness, renal failure, and lower limb amputation. The life expectancy of individuals with type 2 diabetes may be shortened by as much as 15 years, with up to 80% dying of cardiovascular disease (CVD).

The onset of most cases of type 2 diabetes is preceded by a latent phase of glucose intolerance or impaired glucose regulation. Impaired glucose regulation, also termed prediabetes, consists of impaired fasting glucose (IFG) and/or impaired glucose tolerance (IGT). In addition to diabetes itself, IGT and/orIFG also constitutes a cause of major public health concern, both because of their association with diabetes incidence and their association with an increased risk of the development of CVD. Some 70% of individuals with IGT or IFG are expected to develop diabetes by 10–15 years if there are no lifestyle modifications or therapeutic interventions.

According to the International Diabetes Federation (IDF), approximately 285 million (6.4%) people, in the 20–79 year age group had diabetes and 344 million (7.8%) had IGT in 2010. About 70% of these live in low and middle income countries. By 2030, the number of people with diabetes and IGT are projected to increase to 438 million (7.7%) and 472 million (8.4%), respectively [1].

The Western Pacific region with 77 million and the South-East Asian region with 59 million had the largest number of people with diabetes in 2010. By 2030, the diabetes prevalence of all regions will have increased, with near doubling of numbers in Africa, the Middle East, and North Africa. The highest prevalence will continue to be in North America and the Caribbean, the Middle East and North Africa, and South-East Asia [1].

Epidemiologic trends of diabetes in Asian Indians and migrant South Asians

Worldwide international migration is a growing phenomenon. According to the International Organization for Migration (IOM) there are now about 192 million people living outside their place of birth, which is about 3% of the world's population. This means that roughly one in every 35 persons in the world is a migrant. Between 1965 and 1990, the number of international migrants increased by 45 million – an annual growth rate of about 2.1%. The current annual growth rate is about 2.9% [2].

South Asians originate from the Indian sub-continent (India, Pakistan, Bangladesh, Sri Lanka, and Nepal) and represent one-fifth of the world's population. More than 2 million South Asians live in the United States and almost 1 million in Canada. In the United Kingdom, this ethnic group increased rapidly during the last 30 years and currently comprise the largest ethnic minority group, representing 4% of the total population. The majority belong to the lower socioeconomic classes, economically and/or socially, at least in the initial phases of settlement in the country.

In comparison with the prevalence of diabetes in Asian Indians and immigrants living in the same environmental conditions, Asian Indians have excessive risk for type 2 diabetes and other related chronic diseases such as cardiovascular and renal diseases, irrespective of their religion, diet, or socioeconomic status. It occurs at a younger age and at a much lower body mass index (BMI). In Canada, a higher proportion of South Asians (62.5%) were diagnosed prior to age 50 compared with approximately one-third (34.7%) of white people. The mean age at which initial diabetes diagnoses occurred was 44.6 years in South Asians and 51.4 years in white people. In the United Kingdom, prevalence rates of type 2 diabetes are three- to fourfold higher in South Asians than the general population. The age at presentation is also significantly younger, and the condition remains undiagnosed in up to 40% of South Asian individuals. Prevalence rates of type 2 diabetes in migrant South Asians was highest in the United Kingdom (11–33%) followed by Norway (14–28%), the United States (18%), Singapore (12.8%), Canada (10%), and New Zealand (8.3%) [3]; whereas the prevalence for native South Asians in Pakistan, India, and Bangladesh is 7.6%, 7.1%, and 6.1%, respectively (Table 7.1) [1].

The projected increase in regional diabetes prevalence from 7.0% in 2010 to 8.4% in 2030 is very much a consequence of the increasing life expectancy over 50 years, is expected to increase from 16% to 23% between 2010 and 2030, and people residing in urban areas will also increase from 33% to 46% [1]. South Asians living in cities in the subcontinent have much higher rates of type 2 diabetes than rural populations but rates are increasing in both rural and urban areas as lifestyles become more westernized. In 1999, the prevalence of diabetes in rural and urban areas of Bangladesh was 2.3% and 8.8% in various age groups. In India (2004), it was 3.1% and 7.3% in rural and urban areas, respectively, and in Pakistan (1995), it was 6.5% and 10.8% in rural and urban areas, respectively. At the same time, the prevalence rate was several times higher in Bangladeshi and Indian immigrants living in westernized countries.

Risk factors for type 2 diabetes in Asian Indians and migrant South Asians

The exponential rise in type 2 diabetes can be attributed to environmental exposure on the background of genetic susceptibility. Over the last half century there has been rapid socioeconomic development in many countries resulting in a move from a traditional to a modern (urbanization/ westernization) way of life. In virtually all populations, higher fat and lower fiber containing diets and decreased physical activity have accompanied modernization. These changes in diet and physical inactivity,

Table 7.1 Prevalence of type 2 diabetes among Asian Indians and migrant South Asians.

Study design	Year	Setting	Sampling methods	Sample size	M/F	Age (yr)	Population	Diagnostic methods	Prevalence	Reference
Cross-sectional survey [4]	2006–2007	UK	Medical practices with deprived population	34359	26637/17772	>20	SAs, Caucasian & Blacks	Diagnostic read code for T2DM	11 (SAs), 3.5 (Caucasians) 8 (Blacks)	Dreyer et al. [4]
Cross-sectional survey [5]	2001–2003	UK	Random	435	271/164	20–75	Migrant SAs	OGTT	20	Hanif et al. [5]
Population-based study [6]	2001	UK	Random	1063	517/546	35–79	Urban migrant Pakistanis, Europeans & Afro-Caribbeans	OGTT	33 (Pakistanis)[a] 20 (Europeans) 22 (Caribbeans)	Riste et al. [6]
Population-based study [7]	1996–1998	Canada	Stratified from previous survey	985	506/479	35–79	Urban ethnic SAs, Europeans & Chinese	FBG	10 (SAs)[a] 5 (Europeans) 2 (Chinese)	Anand et al. [7]
Community based study [8]	2004	USA	Random	1046	537/509	17–87	Asian Indian migrants	Self-reported	18.3	Venkataraman et al. [8]
Cross-sectional survey [9]	1984–1995	Singapore	Registry from previous surveys	5707	2796/2911	24–64	Asian Indian, Malay, Chinese	FBG	12.8 (Indians)[a] 4 (Malay) 3 (Chinese)	Yeo et al. [9]

(Continued)

Table 7.1 (*Continued*)

Study design	Year	Setting	Sampling methods	Sample size	M/F	Age (yr)	Population	Diagnostic methods	Prevalence	Reference
Population-based study [10]	1992	Singapore	Random	3568	1712/1856	18–69	Asian Indian, Malay, Chinese	OGTT	12.2 (Indians)[a] 10.1 (Malay) 7.8 (Chinese)	Tan et al. [10]
Population cohort. 10-yr follow-up [11]	1994	South Africa	Systemic cluster	563	232/331	>15	South African Indians	OGTT	16.2*	Motala et al. [11]
Cross-sectional survey [12]	2000	Norway	Random	2513	1101/1412	30–67	SAs & western volunteers	Self-reported	14.3/27.5 (SAs)[a,b] 5.9/2.9 (West)[a,b]	Jenum et al. [12]
Population-based study [13]	2003– 2005	India	Stratified	44523	21816/22707	15–64	Rural and urban	Self-reported	4.5 (3.1 & 7.3)	Mohan et al, [13]
Cross-sectional survey [14]	1999– 2002	India	Random	41270	20534/20736	≥25	Rural and urban	FBG	4.3 (1.9 & 4.6)	Sadikot et al, [14]
Cross-sectional survey [15]	1999	Bangladesh	Random	6312	2768/3544	≥20	Rural and urban	FBG and OGTT (selected number)	2.3/8.1	Hussain et al. [15]
Population-based survey [16]	1995	Pakistan	Cluster	1404	435/969	≥25	Rural and urban	OGTT	6.5/10.8	Shera et al. [16]

FBG, fasting blood glucose; OGTT, oral glucose tolerance test; SAs, South Asians.

[a]Adjusted for age and gender.

[b]Values reported as males/females.

combined with increasing longevity and obesity, have formed the basis for dramatic increases in the prevalence of diabetes mellitus both in developed and developing countries.

Various ethnic groups within western populations have pointed out differences in susceptibility to diabetes within the same environmental pressure. There are both economic and ethical reasons for the increasing burden of type 2 diabetes prevalence among immigrants. Ethnicity-related differences in the risk of type 2 diabetes may have been attributable to genetics, epigenetics, fetal, and environmental factors (Forsdahl–Barker hypothesis), and also to the Western lifestyle with reduced physical activity and calorie-dense diet.

Important risk factors for Asian Indians immigrants follow.

Overall and abdominal obesity

According to International Association for the Study of Obesity, more than 1.5 billion adults worldwide are overweight, and 525 million are obese. In addition, at least 155 million children worldwide are overweight or obese [17]. Asians have lower rates of overweight and obesity than their Western counterparts. In India, between 2003 and 2005, the prevalence of overweight ranged from 9.4% in rural men to 38.8% in urban women. Using the same World Health Organization (WHO) BMI cut-point, the prevalence of overweight was 28.6% in urban Pakistan and 26.2% in rural Bangladesh. Despite lower BMI, some Asian countries have similar or even higher prevalence of diabetes than Western countries. Almost 80% of South Asian type 2 diabetic patients are not obese, whereas 60–80% of such diabetics in the West are obese. The build and habitus, far from being overweight, is often "lean" or low body weight (i.e., more than 20% below the ideal body weight for height and sex). About one-quarter of type 2 diabetes patients in India and Bangladesh have BMI below $19 \, kg/m^2$ [18]. The prevalence of lean type 2 diabetes was 3.8% in rural Bangladesh, and in India it varied from 3.5% to 25%. A rural Bangladesh study found a reverse association between relative changes in BMI and incidence of diabetes for those who lost their BMI from initial values and those who gained excessively (Figure 7.1). In general, those who maintained a stable BMI (–5% to +5%) had a lower risk of diabetes which means that obesity alone may not explain the increased occurrence of diabetes in Asian populations. These Asian Indian rural communities may be experiencing a double burden of diabetes epidemics (i.e., obesity-related diabetes among the affluent and undernutrition-related diabetes in the poor).

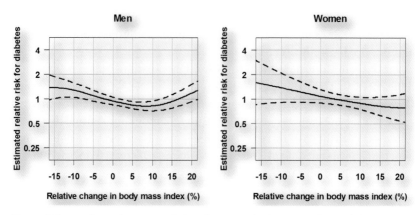

Figure 7.1 Association between relative changes in body mass index and the incidence of diabetes in rural Asian Indian (Asghar et al. [19]).

Asian populations, especially those of South Asian descent, are more prone to abdominal obesity and low muscle mass with increased insulin resistance than their Western counterparts. Thus, waist circumference reflecting central obesity is a useful measure of obesity-related risk of type 2 diabetes, especially in individuals with normal BMI values. For the same age, sex, and BMI, South Asians have a higher percentage of body fat than white Caucasians. In Caucasian men, a BMI of $30\,kg/m^2$ corresponds to 25% body fat [20], whereas in South Asian men, a BMI of $<25\,kg/m^2$ corresponds to 33% body fat [21]. Despite having a lower body weight, Indian infants have higher subcutaneous fat, leptin, and insulin levels than white infants. This "metabolically obese" phenotype (e.g., normal weight by conventional BMI standards but increased abdominal adiposity) has been associated with increased risk of insulin resistance and diabetes. Plasma adiponectin concentrations are lower in South Asians than Caucasians. Thus, reduced adiponectin levels might contribute to the increased risk of type 2 diabetes and CVD in South Asians [22].

Food habits

Intake of dietary energy in excess of expenditure will result in weight gain and, depending on the degree and type of weight gain, increased risk of type 2 diabetes. For each kilogram of weight gain it has been calculated that the risk for diabetes increases by about 4.5%. South Asians consume lower amounts of protein and greater quantities of total fat, monounsaturated fatty acids, eggs, dairy products, and carbohydrates (about 60–70% of energy intake) than Europeans. In addition, frying is a common food preparation method among South Asians.

Vegetable ghee, such as *dalda* – a clarified butter commonly used in cooking in India and other -South-East Asian countries – contains trans fatty acid levels as high as 50%. Higher intake of trans fatty acids has been associated with weight gain, increased cardiometabolic risk, and insulin resistance. Polished rice and refined wheat form the basis of most Asian diets with high glycemic index and glycemic load values. A high intake of foods with a high glycemic index or glycemic load, especially rice, is associated with a twofold increased risk of type 2 diabetes, especially in overweight and obese individuals [18]. Consumption of sugar-sweetened beverages, an important contributor of dietary glycemic load and excess calories, has increased rapidly worldwide, particularly in Asia Indian children. n-3 polyunsaturated fatty acids (PUFA) confer CVD protection through a variety of mechanisms. South Asians show a lower consumption of n-3 PUFA than Europeans [23].

Physical activity

Physical inactivity represents an independent cardiometabolic risk factor and exercise is recommended to control and also prevent diabetes. Regular physical activity reduces the risk of type 2 diabetes in adults by 20–60% in a dose–response manner. Lower physical activity scores have been reported in South Asians than white populations [24,25]. South Asians appear to ignore the beneficial effects of exercise and a lack of guidance from their physicians might partly account for this. Levels of physical activity were inversely associated with BMI, waist circumference, glucose and insulin levels in South Asians.

Developmental origins of diabetes

Fetal undernutrition and being born small for gestational age have been identified as risk factors of type 2 diabetes among both adults and youth. Low birth weight (birth weight <2.5 kg) is a significant etiologic factor in the development of type 2 diabetes. According to the "thrifty phenotype" hypothesis, the combination of being undernourished *in utero* followed by a nutritionally overabundant environment later in life may unmask certain fetally programmed predispositions such as central adiposity, decreased pancreatic beta-cell growth, subnormal insulin secretory responses and insulin receptors functions, and activity of the hypothalamic–pituitary–adrenal axis. These abnormalities, in turn, may increase susceptibility to insulin resistance and type 2 diabetes. Low birth weight and exposure to undernutrition *in utero* are common in some Asian populations, especially in the Indian subcontinent, where 30% of infants are underweight. Prospective studies from India have shown the impact of fetal undernutrition (often manifested as low birth weight) as well as overnutrition (e.g., the infant of a mother with diabetes) on future risk of diabetes. In India, thinness in infancy and overweight at age 12 years was associated with increased risk of developing IGT or diabetes in young adulthood [18].

The two- to threefold higher risk of gestational diabetes in Asian women than in their white counterparts also may contribute to the increasing epidemic of young onset diabetes in Asia. Asian women with a history of gestational diabetes have a substantially increased risk of diabetes, while their offspring exhibit early features of the metabolic syndrome, thus setting up a vicious cycle of "diabetes begetting diabetes." This combination of gestational diabetes, *in utero* nutritional imbalance, childhood obesity, and overnutrition in adulthood will continue to fuel the epidemic in Asian countries undergoing rapid nutritional transitions [18].

Genetic factors

Genetic factors also play an important part in the development of type 2 diabetes, as exemplified by rare monogenic subtypes, the high prevalence in particular ethnic groups, and its modification by genetic admixture and the difference in concordance rates between monozygotic and dizygotic twins. However, the role of genetics in the development of diabetes is poorly understood. Asian Indians are apparently genetically more prone to diabetes and insulin resistance than other ethnic populations. Moreover, Asian Indians are more susceptible to develop truncal obesity, which might account for their tendency to insulin resistance referred to as "Asian Indian phenotype." Most diabetes genetic variants identified so far, including those in *TCF7L2* and *KCNQ1*, appear to be associated with decreased insulin secretion in white people as well as Asians [26]. In addition, among Asian adults diagnosed with diabetes before age 40 years, approximately 40% had a lean nonautoimmune phenotype with rapid oral drug failure. Approximately 10% of these patients carried genetic variants encoding pancreatic beta-cell pathways, including transcription factors and amylin, or mitochondrial polymorphisms. These findings provide further evidence that beta-cell dysfunction has a critical role in the development of diabetes in Asians.

Summary of the identified risk factors

Overweight is the most critical risk factor, and should be targeted for prevention of type 2 diabetes especially among young people. Diet and physical activity, which mediate energy balance, are also clearly related to

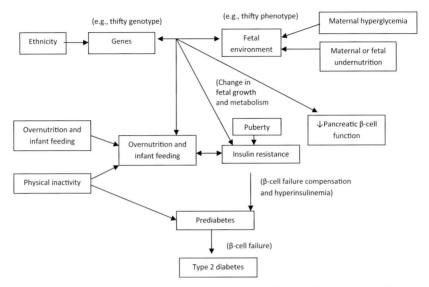

Figure 7.2 Interaction of risk factors for prediabetes and type 2 diabetes (Hussain et al. [27]).

diabetes risk. Ethnicity and perinatal factors (i.e., being born either large or small for gestational age or to a mother with diabetes during pregnancy) may also be risk factors. The risk appears to be of particular importance for certain ethnic groups. Perinatal factors include both nonmodifiable and modifiable risk factors for the development of type 2 diabetes, and therefore should be included in preventive strategies. Nonmodifiable risk factors useful in identifying high-risk young people include family history of type 2 diabetes. The interaction of these factors is shown in Figure 7.2.

Preventive strategies

There are a lack of randomized controlled trials to elucidate to what extent components of type 2 diabetes may be beneficially influenced by a culturally adapted approach, especially among non-Western immigrants living in Western countries. The IDF classifies diabetes prevention into three levels: primary, secondary, and tertiary. Primary intervention includes activities that prevent diabetes from developing. Secondary prevention includes early detection of diabetes, prompt and effective management of diabetes, and also measures to halt its progression. Tertiary prevention includes measures undertaken to prevent complications and physical disabilities brought about by diabetes. Diet, exercise, stress management, and weight control are important at any level of diabetes prevention and treatment. Public health efforts should be encouraged to implement education at a population level and encourage environmental changes to modify the identifiable "diabesogenic" factors of "Western" societies.

To curb this epidemic, an integrated strategy combining population-wide preventive policies (e.g., changing food and the built environment), early detection, and multidisciplinary care programs may reduce the risk of diabetes and associated complications in both the general population and in high-risk individuals. On the basis of modifiable risk factors for type 2 diabetes, many prevention programs have focused on lifestyle modifications, although other strategies including the use of pharmacologic agents, which target either improvement in the beta-cell function or insulin resistance, have also been used. The US Diabetes Prevention Program (DPP) had three arms in the study: placebo, metformin, and intensive lifestyle changes. After an average follow-up of 2.8 years, there was a 58% relative reduction in the progression to diabetes in the lifestyle group compared with the control group. Within this group, 50% achieved the goal of more than 7% weight reduction, and 74% maintained at least 150 minutes of moderately intense activity each week. It is interesting that the Indian Diabetes Prevention Programme (IDPP) showed that diabetes played a significant role of moderate lifestyle modification even without significant weight reduction (Table 7.2 and Table 7.3).

There are a lack of intervention studies focusing on the physiologic and psychologic aspects of the blood glucose regulation [43]. However, as yet, there have not been any large-scale lifestyle studies on immigrant populations.

It is well known that antidiabetic drugs only have a limited effect on type 2 diabetes, and there is reliable evidence showing good associations between lifestyle factors such as dietary habits, body weight, and physical activity, and the incidence of type 2 diabetes. Lifestyle intervention has been shown to prevent type 2 diabetes [43], but studies in immigrants are scarce. At an international level, large-scale interventions have been conducted and proven successful in changing diet and physical activity to prevent type 2 diabetes (Table 7.2). Similar interventions have been carried out in different cultures, but with local ethnic groups not immigrants.

Unfortunately, many immigrants are not reached by national public health programs, for reasons of language problems and different cultural

Table 7.2 Summary of studies involving lifestyle (diet and exercise) interventions.

Study	Number of people	Years of follow-up	Mean age and mean BMI	Type of intervention	Frequency of intervention	Targets	Effect of intervention
Malmo, Sweden [28,29]	181 (men only)	6.0	48 years 26 kg/m^2	Diet, exercise	Monthly for 6/12, then every 12/12	Unspecified weight loss	Reduction in diabetes incidence in intervention group 37% 2.0–3.3 kg weight loss
Da Qing, China [30]	577	6.0	45 years 25.6 kg/m^2	Diet, exercise, or both	7 sessions in 3/12, then every 3/12	BMI <23 kg/m^2, healthier diet	Reduction in diabetes incidence per group: 31%
DPS, Finland [31]	522	3.2	55 years 31 kg/m^2	Diet, exercise	7 sessions in 12/12, then every 3/12 Free gym membership and supervised activity sessions	5% weight loss, decrease fat intake, increase fiber intake >150 min exercise/week	Reduction in diabetes incidence in intervention group – 58% (63% in men and 54% in women) 3.5 kg weight loss after 2 years
New Zealand [32]	103	5.0	52 years 29 kg/m^2	Diet	Monthly for first 12/12	Unspecified weight loss, reduced fat intake	No benefit in progression to diabetes No weight loss
Malmohus, Sweden [33]	267 (men only)	10.0	54.1 years (mean weight 76 kg)	Diet and exercise	Every 12/12		Reduction in diabetes – 13% diet group, 29% control, no weight loss
FHS [34]	188	6.0	50 years (mean weight 81.7 kg)	Diet, exercise	Every 3/12	Lose weight if BMI >22 kg/m^2, low fat diet, exercise 3–4 times/week	No benefit in progression to diabetes No weight loss
DPP, USA [35]	3234	2.8	51 years, 34 kg/m^2	Diet, exercise	16 diet sessions in 6/12, then monthly. Twice- weekly supervised exercise sessions	7% weight loss, low-fat diet, 150 min exercise/ week	Decreased progression to diabetes per group 58% diet and exercise 3.8 kg weight loss
Indian Diabetes Prevention Program (IDPP) [36]	531	3.0	45.9 years 25.8 kg/m^2	Diet and exercise, Metformin, Diet, exercise and metformin	6 months interval	Unspecified weight loss, reduce calorie and fat intake, moderate physical activity	Reduction in diabetes incidence in LSM –28.5% Met group –26.4% LSM + Met –28.2%
DPP, Japan [37]	304	3.0	51 years 23 kg/m^2	Diet, exercise	Every 3/12 then 6/12	5% weight loss, increase leisure time physical activity –700 kcal/week	Reduction in diabetes incidence –53%

Table 7.3 Summary of studies involving lifestyle interventions with oral antidiabetic agents.

Study	Number of people	Inclusion criteria	Years of fol-low up	Mean age and mean BMI	Oral antidiabetic agent	Type of intervention	Frequency of intervention	Specified targets other than to delay progression to diabetes	Effect of intervention
Malmohus, Sweden [38]	267 (men only)	IGT using a 30-g glucose/m² body surface area OGTT: 1-h glc > 8.9, 2-h glc > 6.7 or 3-h glc > 4.7 mmol/L	10	54.1 years (mean weight 76 kg)	Tolbutamide	Diet, exercise, weight loss	Every 12/12	–	Decreased progression to diabetes per group; 29%. No weight loss
Whitehall [39]	200	2-h glucose value after 50-g OGTT 6.7–11.0 mmol/L	5	56 years 26.2 kg/m²	Phenformin	Carbohydrate restricted diet	Once at start of study	Unspecified weight loss	No benefit in progression to diabetes, weight loss 1.2 kg
FHS [40]	188	Fasting glucose 5.5–7.7 mmol/L	6	50 years (mean weight 81.7 kg)	Gliclazide	Diet, exercise	Every 3/12	Lose weight if BMI >22 kg/m², low fat diet, exercise 3–4 times/week	No benefit in progression to diabetes, no weight loss

Study	n	Inclusion criteria	Duration (years)	Age/BMI	Intervention	Comparison	Frequency	Intervention details	Outcomes
DPP, USA [35,41,42]	3234	IGT + fasting glucose > 5.3 mmol/L. 45% ethnic minority	2.8	51 years 34 kg/m²	Metformin	Diet, exercise	16 diet sessions in 6/12, then monthly. Twice weekly supervised exercise sessions	7% weight loss, low-fat diet, 150 min exercise/week	Decreased progression to diabetes per group; 58% diet and exercise (71% in people aged >70) >metformin. 3.8 kg weight loss diet + exercise. 1.8 kg weight loss metformin
STOP NIDDM [32,33]	1429	IGT + fasting glucose > 5.6 mmol/L	3.3	55 years 31 kg/m²	Acarbose	General advice on diet, weight loss and activity.	Every 12/12	–	Acarbose decreased progression to diabetes by 25%. Weight loss 0.5 kg
EDIT [35,38]	631	Fasting glucose 5.5–7.7 mmol/L	6	52 years 28.6 kg/m²	Metformin, acarbose or both	None	Unspecified	–	In patients with IGT at baseline, decreased risk of progression to diabetes with acarbose, no weight loss
IDPP [36]	531	Fasting glucose < 7.0 mmol/L 2 hr glucose 7.8–11.0 mmol/L	3	45.9 years 25.8 kg/m²	Metformin	Diet and exercise Metformin Diet, exercise, and metformin	6 month interval	Unspecified weight loss Reduce calorie and fat intake Moderate physical activity	Reduction in diabetes incidence in LSM −28.5% Met −26.4% LSM + Met −28.2%

perceptions on health and disease. Health personnel tend to view the immigrant population as a particularly challenging group [44]. There are both economic and ethical reasons for trying to attenuate the burden of type 2 diabetes prevalence among immigrants, and to smooth out the inequalities in health.

The InnaDiab DE-PLAN study [45] has taken the factors discussed below into the nondirective cultural approach in a randomized controlled trial on Pakistani women living in Norway, with focus on post meal blood glucose regulation for preventing type 2 diabetes, in line with the recommendations of the IDF (www.IDF.com 2011). The InnaDiab DE-PLAN study aimed to follow the principles of nondirective support [46], emphasizing information rather than communication of rules of conduct. Instead of detailed diet advice, the participants were encouraged to apply the knowledge in their own way, in order to acquire personal control of their lifestyle. The main focus in the intervention group was the physiologic importance of blood glucose and its regulation. All education sessions emphasized the importance of blood glucose and its control for preventing type 2 diabetes. Information on the blood glucose and insulin raising effect of simple sugars and starch was repeated, as was the strong blunting effect of light post meal physical activity.

The main principle is that nondirective support may be helpful when the individual has acquired a positive approach to his/her ability to cope. This may be particularly important for immigrants trying to find their way in a new and challenging cultural environment. If this is true, we expected that this modification of an information program would have positive effects on attendance, behavior, and ultimately on physiology and other risk factors for type 2 diabetes. Most of the participants in the study had not reached that level of pathology at baseline. However, the rapid development of the disorder in the control group during the 7 months' intervention period was alarming. At 3-year follow-up the results were surprisingly good, with many of the important risk factors for type 2 diabetes improving even more than after 1 year post test.

This is in line with Hawthorne et al. [47] who showed similar results from a diabetes health education program for British Pakistani women. Kousar et al. [48] showed that a culturally adopted lifestyle intervention in Pakistani women reduced the risk factors for metabolic syndrome.

A nondirective approach to advice given may therefore be particularly important for this group [49]. The important principle is to provide balanced information rather than imposing the counselor's values on the client. There is, of course, no clearcut boundary between directive and nondirective advice [50]. For diabetic patients, it has been shown that nondirective social support is associated with better metabolic control, at least for young patients. Directive support appears to be counterproductive [51].

The IMAGE group has published an evidence-based guideline for prevention of type 2 diabetes [52]. This guideline together with a toolkit [53] give us all we need for preventing the type 2 diabetes in all part of the world, in all nations and for all cultures. We have the facts, we have the evidence, and we have the toolkit so – the time to act is now.

Conclusions

There is a rising need among professionals and policy makers to focus on prevention of type 2 diabetes. Upstream interventions have the potential for making the largest impact on diabetes. However, it is unlikely that a study would ever be undertaken to demonstrate an impact of upstream intervention on the incidence of diabetes or cardiovascular outcomes. It is difficult in the sense of logistics, economy, and ethics to replicate randomized controlled trials in the general population over a prolonged period of time. The most beneficial population-based measures are increased physical activity and decreased consumption of energy-dense foods. This needs combined efforts from governments and research organizations to make the necessary sustainable changes in food consumption and education policy, models of which has been shown to work in Finland. Midstream interventions need to be developed further and evaluated, particularly those that target school children and young people. Other interventions involving ethnic groups, women with gestational diabetes, and obese subjects appear to be promising. The clearest evidence of benefit is in downstream interventions. Targeting those patients with IGT with lifestyle and interventions focused on increasing activity and altering dietary factors has been particularly effective in North American and Finnish populations. Similar results have been obtained in Asian populations.

Migration has become a key part of our collective social and economic development. It is essential that the design of preventative policy and the training of health care practitioners take into account the health of migrants and the challenges posed by conditions such as diabetes. It is equally essential to work with migrants to ensure that they are aware of the possibilities for care and the risks they are exposed to.

References

1. International Diabetes Federation. Diabetes Atlas, 4th edn.
2. International Organization for Migration (IOM). Available from: www.iom.int (accessed 5 March 2013).
3. Garduno SD, Khokhar S. Prevalence, risk factors and complications associated with type 2 diabetes in migrant South Asians. Diabetes Metab Res Rev 2012;28:6–24.
4. Dreyer G, Hull S, Aitken Z, Chesser A, Yaqoob MM. The effect of ethnicity on the prevalence of diabetes and associated chronic kidney disease. Int J Med 2009;102: 261–9.
5. Hanif MW, Valsamakis G, Dixon A, Boutsiadis A, Jones AF, Barnett AH, et al. Detection of impaired glucose tolerance and undiagnosed type 2 diabetes in UK South Asians: an effective screening strategy. Diabetes Obes Metab 2008;10(9):755–62.
6. Riste L, Khan F, Cruickshank K. High prevalence of type 2 diabetes in all ethnic groups, including Europeans, in a British inner city. Diabetes Care 2001;24(8): 1377–83.
7. Anand SS, Yusuf S, Vuksan V, Devanesen S, Teo KK, Montague PA, et al. Differences in risk factors, atherosclerosis, and cardiovascular disease betweed ethnic groups in Canada: the study of health assessment and risk in ethnic groups. Lancet 2000; 356(9226):279–84.
8. Venkataraman R, Nanda NC, Baweja G, Parikh N, Bhatia V. Prevalence of diabetes mellitus and related conditions in Asian Indians living in the United States. Am J Cardiol 2004;94(7):977.
9. Yeo KK, Tai BC, Heng D, Lee JM, Ma S, Hughes K, et al. Ethnicity modifies the association between diabetes mellitus and ischaemic heart disease in Chinese, Malays and Asian Indians living in Singapore. Diabetologia 2006;49(12):2866–73.
10. Tan CE, Emmanuel SC, Tan BY, Jacob E. Prevalence of diabetes and ethnic differences in cardiovascular risk factors: The 1992 Singapore National Health Survey. Diabetes Care 1999;22(2):241–7.
11. Motala AA, Omar MAK, Pirie FJ. Epidemiology of type 1 and type 2 diabetes in Africa. J Cardiovasc Risk 2003;10(2):77–83.
12. Jenum AK, Holme I, Graff-Iversen S, Birkeland KI. Ethnicity and sex are strong determinants of diabetes in an urban Western society: implications for prevention. Diabetologia 2005;48:435–9.
13. Mohan V, Mathur P, Deepa R, Deepa M, Shukla DK, Menon GR, et al. Urban rural differences in prevalence of self-reported diabetes in India: The WHO-ICMR Indian NCD risk factor surveillance. Diabetes Res Clin Pract 2008;80:159–68.
14. Sadikot SM, Nigam A, Das Bajaj S, et al. Comparing the ADA 1997 and the WHO 1999 criteria: Prevalence of diabetes in India Study. Diabetes Res Clin Pract 2004;66(3):309–15.
15. Hussain A, Rahim MA, Khan AK, Ali SMK. Type 2 diabetes in rural and urban population: diverse prevalence and associated risk factors in Bangladesh. Diabetes Med 2005;22:931–7.
16. Shera AS, Rafique G, Khawaja IA, Baqai S, King H. Pakistan National Diabetes Survey: prevalence of glucose intolerance and associated factors in Baluchistan province. Diabetes Res Clin Pract 1999;44(1):49–58.

17. International Association for the Study of Obesity. Available from: www.iaso.org (accessed 5 March 2013).

18. Chan JC, Malik V, Jia W, Kadowaki T, Yajnik CS, Yoon KH, et al. Diabetes in Asia: epidemiology, risk factors, and pathophysiology. JAMA 2009;301(20):2129–40.

19. Asghar S, Hussain A, Khan AK, Ali SM, Sayeed MA, Bhowmik B, et al. Incidence of diabetes in Asian-Indian subjects: a five year follow-up study from Bangladesh. Prim Care Diabetes 2011;5(2):117–24.

20. Dudeja V, Misra A, Pandey RM, Devina G, Kumar G, Vikram NK. BMI does not accurately predict overweight in Asian Indians in northern India. Br J Nutr 2001;86:105–12.

21. Banerji MA, Faridi N, Atluri R, Chaiken RL, Lebovitz HE. Body composition, visceral fat, leptin, and insulin resistance in Asian Indian men. J Clin Endocrinol Metab 1999;84:137–44.

22. Retnakaran R, Hanley AJ, Zinman B. Does hypoadiponectinemia explain the increased risk of diabetes and cardiovascular disease in South Asians? Diabetes Care 2006;29:1950–4.

23. Lovegrove JA, Lovegrove SS, Lesauvage SVM, Brady LM, Saini N, Minihane AM, et al. Moderate fishoil supplementation reverses low-platelet, long-chain n-3 poly-unsaturated fatty acid status and reduces plasma triacylglycerol concentrations in British Indo-Asians. Am J Clin Nutr 2004;79:974–82.

24. Fischbacher CM, Hunt S, Alexander L. How physically active are South Asians in the United Kingdom? A literature review. J Public Health (Oxf) 2004;26:250–8.

25. Hayes L, White M, Unwin N, Bhopal R, Fischbacher C, Harland J, et al. Patterns of physical activity and relationship with risk markers for cardiovascular disease and diabetes in Indian, Pakistani, Bangladeshi and European adults in a UK population. J Public Health Med 2002;24:170–8.

26. Chang YC, Chang TJ, Jiang YD, Kuo SS, Lee KC, Chiu KC, et al. Association study of the genetic polymorphisms of the transcription factor 7-like 2 (TCF7L2) gene and type 2 diabetes in the Chinese population. Diabetes 2007;56(10):2631–7.

27. Hussain A, Claussen B, Ramachandran A, Williams R. Prevention of type 2 diabetes: a review. Diabetes Res Clin Pract 2007;76(3):317–26.

28. Dyson PA, Hammersley MS, Morris RJ, Holman RR, Turner RC, Fasting Hypergly-caemia Study Group. The Fasting Hyperglycaemia Study: II. Randomized controlled trial of reinforced healthy-living advice in subjects with increased but not diabetic fasting plasma glucose. Metabolism 1997;46:50–5.

29. Diabetes Prevention Program Research Group. The Diabetes Prevention Program, Baseline characteristics of the randomized cohort. Diabetes Care 2000;23:1619–29.

30. Diabetes Prevention Program Research Group. Costs associated with the primary prevention of type 2 diabetes mellitus in the diabetes prevention program. Diabetes Care 2003;26:36–47.

31. Chiasson JL, Gomis R, Hanefeld M, Josse RG, Karasik A, Laakso M; STOP-NIDDM Trial Research Group. The STOP-NIDDM Trial: an international study on the efficacy of an α-glucosidase inhibitor to prevent type 2 diabetes in a population with impaired glucose tolerance: rationale, design, and preliminary data. Diabetes Care 1998;21:1720–5.

32. Chiasson JL, Josse RG, Gomis R, Hanefeld M, Karasik A, Laakso M. Acarbose for prevention of type 2 diabetes mellitus: The STOP-NIDDM randomised trial. Lancet 2002;359:2072–7.

33. Hanefeld M, Josse RG, Gomis R, Karasik A, Laakso M, Chiasson JL. Efficacy of acarbose to prevent type 2 diabetes is different in subgroups of subjects with impaired glucose tolerance: The STOP-NIDDM trial. Diabetologia 2002;45:104–5.
34. Chiasson J, Josse RG, Gomis R, Hanefeld M, Karasik A, Laakso M. Acarbose can prevent type 2 diabetes and cardiovascular disease in subjects with impaired glucose tolerance: the STOP-NIDDM trial. Diabetologia 2002;45:104.
35. Holman RR, North BU, Tunbridge FKE. Possible prevention of type 2 diabetes with acarbose or metformin. Diabetes Med 2000;17(Suppl 1):17.
36. Ramachandran A, Snehalatha C, Mary S, Mukesh B, Bhaskar AD, Vijay V. The Indian Diabetes Prevention Programme shows that lifestyle modification and metformin prevent type 2 diabetes in Asian Indian subjects with impaired glucose tolerance (IDPP-1). Diabetologia 2006;49:289–97.
37. Sakane N, Sato J, Tsushita K, Tsujii S, Kotani K, Tsuzaki K, et al. Prevention of type 2 diabetes in a primary healthcare setting: three-year results of lifestyle intervention in Japanese subjects with impaired glucose tolerance. BMC Public Health 2011;11(1):40.
38. Holman RR, Blackwell L, Stratton IM, Manley SE, Tucker L, Frighi V. Six-year results from the Early Diabetes Intervention Trial. Diabetes Med 2003;20:S15.
39. Azen SP, Peters RK, Berkowitz K, Kjos S, Xiang A, Buchanan TA. TRIPOD (TROglitazone In the Prevention of Diabetes): a randomized, placebo-controlled trial of troglitazone in women with prior gestational diabetes mellitus. Control Clin Trials 1998;19:217–31.
40. Sjostrom L, Torgerson JS, Hauptman J, Boldrin M. XENDOS (XENical in the prevention of Diabetes in Obese Subjects): a landmark study. 9th International Congress on Obesity, 2002, Sao Paulo, Brazil, 2002.
41. Davies MJ, Tringham JR, Troughton J, Khunti KK. Prevention of type 2 diabetes mellitus: a review of the evidence and its application in a UK setting. Diabet Med 2004;21(5):403–14.
42. Ritchie LD, Ganapathy S, Woodward-Lopez G, Gerstein DE, Fleming SE. Prevention of type 2 diabetes in youth: etiology, promising interventions and recommendations. Pediatr Diabetes 2003;4(4):174–209.
43. Tuomilehto J. Nonpharmacologic therapy and exercise in the prevention of type 2 diabetes. Diabetes Care 2009;32(Suppl 2):189–93.
44. Hussain-Gambles M, Leese B, Atkin K, Brown J, Mason S, Tovey P. Involving South Asian patients in clinical trials. Health Technol Assess 2004;8(42):iii, 1–109.
45. Hjellset VT. A culturally adapted lifestyle intervention with main focus on blood glucose regulation improved the risk profile for type 2 diabtes in pakistani immigrant women: they are not aliens. Faculty of Medicine, University of Oslo; 2011.
46. Fisher EB Jr, La Greca AM, Greco P, Arfken C, Schneiderman N. Directive and nondirective social support in diabetes management. Int J Behav Med 1997;4(2):131–44.
47. Hawthorne K. Effect of culturally appropriate health education on glycaemic control and knowledge of diabetes in British Pakistani women with type 2 diabetes mellitus. Health Educ Res 2001;16(3):373–81.
48. Kousar R, Burns C, Lewandowski P. A culturally appropriate diet and lifestyle intervention can successfully treat the components of metabolic syndrome in female Pakistani immigrants residing in Melbourne, Australia. Metabolism 2008;57(11):1502–8.

49. Fisher EB, Earp JA, Maman S, Zolotor A. Cross-cultural and international adaptation of peer support for diabetes management. Fam Pract 2010;27(Suppl 1):i 6–16.
50. Williams C, Alderson P, Farsides B. Is nondirectiveness possible within the context of antenatal screening and testing? Soc Sci Med 2002;54:339–47.
51. Fisher EB, Thorpe CT, Devellis BM, Devellis RF. Healthy coping, negative emotions, and diabetes management: a systematic review and appraisal. Diabetes Educ 2007; 33(6):1080–103.
52. Paulweber B, Valensi P, Lindstrom J, Lalic NM, Greaves CJ, McKee M, et al. A European evidence-based guideline for the prevention of type 2 diabetes. Horm Metab Res 2010;42(Suppl 1):3–36.
53. Lindstrom J, Neumann A, Sheppard KE, Gilis-Januszewska A, Greaves CJ, Handke U, et al. Take action to prevent diabetes: the IMAGE toolkit for the prevention of type 2 diabetes in Europe. Horm Metab Res 2010;42(Suppl 1):S37–55.

CHAPTER 8

Diabetes prevention in practice: examples from the real world

Konstantinos Makrilakis[1], Stavros Liatis[1], Aleksandra Gilis-Januszewska[2] and Peter Schwarz[3]

[1] First Department of Propaedeutic Medicine, Athens University Medical School, Laiko General Hospital, Athens, Greece
[2] Department of Endocrinology, Collegium Medicum, Jagiellonian University, Krakow, Poland
[3] Department of Medicine III, University of Dresden, Dresden, Germany

Introduction

The frequency of type 2 diabetes (T2D) is increasing worldwide and is reaching epidemic proportions, linked with the aging of the population, a sedentary lifestyle, and a rise in obesity [1]. Furthermore, it is estimated that approximately one-third of all people with diabetes may be undiagnosed [2]. People with T2D have a two to four times higher risk of cardiovascular disease (CVD) and their life expectancy is lower than the rest of the population. Premature mortality caused by diabetes results in an estimated 12–14 years of life lost [3]. The economic burden of treating diabetes and its complications is likewise enormous [4]. As a result, it is imperative that effective primary prevention programs for T2D are urgently instituted, to reduce the clinical and economic health burden.

T2D is characterized by a long prediabetic period [5]. Many controlled clinical trials have shown that intervention at the prediabetic state, either with lifestyle modification [6,7] or with medications [8,9], can prevent, or at least delay, the progression of the disease (for an extensive review see [10]). Lifestyle intervention is the preferred mode of action to prevent diabetes and no medication so far has been approved by authorities or has been recommended by scientific organizations (with the exception of metformin in certain very high-risk individuals) [10,11]. However, randomized controlled trials, with individual counseling usually lasting several years, are expensive and their applicability in the "real life" setting is not always feasible [12,13].

There is a clear consensus at EU level that immediate action is needed to develop targeted prevention programs for T2D [14,15]. A project proposal was submitted by the Department of Public Health, University of Helsinki, to the European Commission, in 2004 (DE-PLAN, Diabetes in Europe – Prevention using Lifestyle, Physical Activity and Nutritional Intervention). The major aim of the project was to establish a model for the efficient identification of individuals at high risk for T2D in EU member countries and also to test the feasibility and cost-effectiveness of the translation of the intervention concepts learned from the prevention trials into existing health care systems [16].

The purpose of this chapter is to present the experience of the efforts to implement a community-based lifestyle intervention program for T2D prevention in Greece and Poland, under real world settings, and describe their effectiveness in preventing the disease.

The Greek experience

The project in Greece was exclusively based on the DE-PLAN study. The setting of the study was in the outpatient domain, in particular in primary health care centers and in occupational settings. The target population comprised all adults aged 35–70 years, without known diabetes who resided in the metropolitan area of Athens.

The previously validated Finnish Type 2 Diabetes Risk Score (FINDRISC) questionnaire [17] was used to identify high-risk individuals for the development of T2D. This is comprised of eight items and a score ≥15 (out of a maximum 26) was considered as the threshold for identification of those at high risk.

As there had been no previous diabetes prevention programs in Greece, this project started from scratch. The strategy used to distribute the FINDRISC questionnaires was variable. An initial effort to distribute the questionnaires to the general population using flyers at health fair events for the public was met with failure (only a minority of questionnaires were filled in). Advertisements for research purposes in the media are not allowed in Greece and so the only way left was through contact with primary care and various occupational settings (Figure 8.1). The process varied considerably among these study sites.

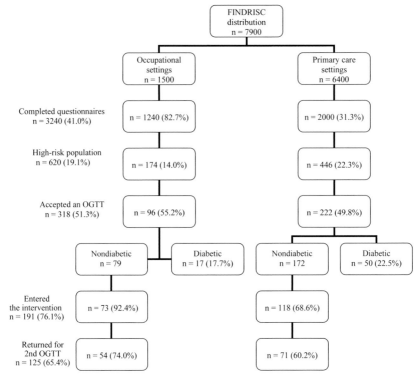

Figure 8.1 Greece: flowchart of the various phases of the project, with number of FINDRISC questionnaires distribution, recruitment of persons at the occupational and primary care setting, and follow-up interventions.

In particular, the medical and nursing staff of six primary care centers, in and around the city of Athens, were contacted and asked to distribute the FINDRISC questionnaires to all people without diabetes visiting their centers, aged 35–70 years Extra leaflets were handed out to be distributed to relatives or friends. People were asked to return the filled-in questionnaires at their next visit. Although the response rate was not *exactly* measured, it was reported by these physicians and nurses to be low – around 30% (Figure 8.1).

In occupational settings, the process of FINDRISC distribution was different. In collaboration with the medical department of six companies in Athens (the Hellenic Telecommunications Company, the Hellenic Radio-television (two sites), the Bank of Greece, an electric equipment manufacturer, and a university hospital), a "Day for diabetes prevention" was arranged at each company. On that day, physicians from the investigators' team visited the company and distributed the FINDRISC questionnaires to all employees attending their job on that specific date. The response rate was substantially higher (around 80%).

In total, 3240 (out of around 7900 distributed) completed FINDRISC questionnaires were collected (Figure 8.1) and 620 high-risk individuals (based on a FINDRISC score ≥15) were identified. All these individuals were invited to have an oral glucose tolerance test (OGTT), in order to exclude people with unknown diabetes. Those without diabetes were then to be followed in the intervention project. A total of 318 participants accepted an OGTT. A positive response to take an OGTT (318/620) was significantly associated with younger age.

During the OGTT, all individuals were asked to fill in a questionnaire regarding their nutritional and physical activity habits. Weight, height, waist circumference, and blood pressure were measured and the medical history recorded.

The project was approved by the cooperating hospital's ethics committee, and the National Drug Organization. All participants signed an informed consent form according to the general recommendations of the Declaration of Helsinki [18].

The 318 OGTT revealed 67 (21.1%) participants with unknown diabetes. Out of the remaining 251 high-risk individuals, 191 (76.1%) agreed to participate in the intervention (Figure 8.1). After the OGTT results, participation in the intervention program (191/251) was no more associated with age (odds ratio (OR) for the highest vs. the lowest quartile 0.94, 95% CI 0.42–2.11), but with the presence of any degree of dysglycemia (OR for the presence of IFG, IGT, or both 2.53, 95% CI 1.40–4.54), and the recruitment from an occupational rather than a primary care setting (OR 4.90, 95% CI 2.12–11.35).

The 1-year intervention program consisted of six sessions (1 hour each) held by a registered dietitian near the participant's residence or work (depending on the recruitment setting). Groups of 6–10 people were formed and each group met with the same dietitian every 2 months.

The nutritional intervention program included the following.
1. Thematic interactive lectures on various nutritional subjects, related to diabetes (e.g., types and sources of carbohydrates, types of dietary fats, nutritional value of vegetables and fruits, importance of fiber).
2. Food intake recording as a method to detect common nutritional mistakes in practice.
3. Provision of specific leaflets and nutritional information on topics such as the diet during Christmas or summer holidays, the caloric content

of foods and snacks, lists of low-fat products (e.g., low-fat cheese), and the importance of olive oil.
4. Weight reducing dietary programs, based on the usual dietary meal plan and food habits of the people attending the program.
5. Food score tests on obesity, CVD risk, general knowledge on nutrition and diabetes.
6. Discussion on common Greek recipes and how to decrease the fat caloric content.

It must be noted that no formal exercise sessions were provided, except for general counseling to increase physical activity.

One-year results and evaluation of the program

Table 8.1 shows the baseline data. Adherence to the intervention sessions varied considerably (15.7% attended only one session, 12.6% completed two, 13.6% three, 13.1% four, 19.4% five, and 25.7% all six sessions). In univariate analysis, higher adherence (four visits or more) was associated with younger age, male sex, recruitment from an occupational rather than a primary health center, and having a higher educational level. In a mul-

Table 8.1 Greece: Baseline data of the initial cohort (mean ± SD).

Variable	Total	Primary care centers	Occupational centers
Number (% males)	191 (40%)	118 (31%)	73 (55%)
Age (years)	56.3 (10.8)	51.3 (9.2)	59.4 (10.6)
FINDRISC Diabetes Risk Score	17.5 (2.4)	17.6 (2.5)	17.5 (2.4)
Weight (kg)	88.7 (14.2)	87.6 (14.2)	90.4 (14.1)
BMI (kg/m²)	32.3 (5.0)	32.9 (5.7)	31.5 (3.7)
Waist circumference (cm)	103.0 (11.3)	108.9 (11.3)	108.5 (9.5)
Males (n = 77)	108.7 (10.3)	98.8 (10.8)	100.0 (9.2)
Females (n = 114)	99.1 (10.3)		
Current smokers (%)	30.0	24.6	37.0
Blood pressure (mmHg)	132/79	133/77	129/82
Glucose fasting plasma (mmol/L)	5.79 (0.64)	5.8 (0.6)	5.7 (0.6)
Glucose 2 hr post-load OGTT (mmol/L)	6.65 (1.81)	7.0 (1.8)	6.1 (1.8)
Cholesterol (mmol/L)	5.80 (0.96)	5.80 (0.9)	5.70 (1.0)
Triglycerides (mmol/L)	1.44 (0.74)	1.5 (0.8)	1.4 (0.7)
HDL-C (mmol/L)	1.28 (0.21)	1.3 (0.2)	1.2 (0.2)
LDL-C (mmol/L)	3.87 (0.88)	3.9 (0.9)	3.9 (0.9)

BMI, body mass index; HDL-C, high density lipoprotein cholesterol; LDL-C, low density lipoprotein cholesterol; OGTT, oral glucose tolerance test.

tivariate logistic regression model, only recruitment from an occupational center ($P = 0.004$) and male sex ($P = 0.007$) were significantly associated with higher compliance to the intervention visits.

A repeat OGTT was performed on 125 (65%) of the participants at the end of 1 year. The reasons for not showing up for a second OGTT were not clear. The majority (55–60%) claimed that they found the procedure unpleasant and time-consuming. Nonreturners were more likely to be women than men (46/114 vs. 19/77; $P = 0.02$). Occupational centers showed a higher rate of 1-year return (55/73 (75.3%) vs. 71/118 (60.2%)) than primary care centers, $P = 0.03$. It should also be noted that the mean number of attended visits was 2.6 for nonreturners, compared to 4.5 for those who completed their second OGTT evaluation ($P < 0.001$), thus showing that, in general, participation in the program was fairly good [19].

Table 8.2 shows anthropometric and clinical data at baseline and 1 year after the intervention. Weight loss averaged (mean ± SD) 1.0 ± 4.7 kg ($P = 0.022$). Favorable changes were observed for body mass index (BMI), systolic blood pressure, fasting plasma glucose, total and low density lipoprotein (LDL) cholesterol levels.

Weight loss was significant only in participants who completed 4–6 intervention sessions (1.1 ± 4.8 kg, $P = 0.028$ vs. 0.6 ± 4.6 kg for 1–3 sessions, $P =$ NS). In addition, those with impaired fasting glucose (IFG) and/or impaired glucose tolerance (IGT) at baseline lost more weight

Table 8.2 Greece: Anthropometric and clinical data of the participants at baseline and 1 year after the intervention (mean ± SD) (n = 125).

Characteristic	Baseline	1 year after	Difference	P[a]
Weight (kg)	89.0 (13.4)	88.0 (13.6)	1.0 (4.7)	0.022
BMI (kg/m^2)	32.0 (4.3)	31.6 (4.0)	0.5 (2.1)	0.014
Waist circumference (cm)	102.9 (11.0)	102.6 (10.6)	0.3 (6.8)	NS
BP (mmHg)	133/79	127/80	6/–1	<0.001 (for systolic BP)
Glucose fasting (mmol/L)	5.81 (0.63)	5.66 (0.63)	0.15 (0.69)	0.017
Glucose 2 hr (mmol/L)	6.56 (1.79)	6.59 (2.01)	−0.03 (1.85)	NS
Total cholesterol (mmol/L)	5.90 (0.88)	5.53 (0.95)	0.37 (0.99)	<0.0001
Triglycerides (mmol/L)	1.44 (0.82)	1.47 (0.86)	−0.03 (0.68)	NS
HDL-C (mmol/L)	1.29 (0.22)	1.29 (0.21)	0.00 (0.07)	NS
LDL-C (mmol/L)	3.99 (0.79)	3.60 (0.92)	0.39 (0.91)	<0.0001

BMI, body mass index; BP, blood pressure; HDL-C, high density lipoprotein cholesterol; LDL-C, low density lipoprotein cholesterol; NS, nonsignificant.
[a]Comparison between baseline and 1 year data.

(1.5 ± 4.8 kg, $P = 0.005$) than those with normal glucose tolerance (NGT) (gained 0.2 ± 4.5 kg, P = NS).

Glucose dysregulation showed favorable changes with the intervention. The percentage of NGT people increased from 32.0% (40/125) to 40.8% (51/125), while that of dysglycemia decreased significantly from 68.0% (85/125) to 53.6% (67/125). A total of seven people (5.6%) developed diabetes.

The dietary aims of the intervention were combined to form a scoring system (intervention's dietary scoring system; IDS score) and this score was used to evaluate the participants' dietary habits both at baseline and at the end of the intervention. An increase in the score was considered to reflect favorable changes, according to the intervention's goals [20].

At the end of the intervention, individuals significantly decreased whole fat dairy products, processed meat consumption (P = 0.018 and 0.016, respectively), sugars (P = 0.006), and refined cereals intake (P = 0.045), whereas fruits and vegetables intake, as well as total time spent daily on physical activity, did not change significantly. The IDS increased significantly, indicating an overall improvement of the dietary habits at the end of the intervention (15.8 ± 2.9 at baseline vs. 16.6 ± 3.1 1 year later, $P < 0.001$). The increase in the IDS was associated with weight loss (r = 0.209, P = 0.021) indicating that individuals with greater dietary improvement experienced greater weight loss [20]. It was found that 58.7% of the participants improved their diet, 33.9% reported worse dietary habits, and 7.4% reported unchanged dietary habits. Compared with baseline, those individuals who improved their diet reduced their body weight (P = 0.007), BMI (P = 0.005), total cholesterol (P = 0.002), and fasting plasma glucose levels ($P = 0.027$). On the contrary, those whose diets worsened had no significant changes in the respective anthropometric and clinical indices compared with baseline.

The Polish experience

In Poland, the DE-PLAN Krakow project was carried out in an urban setting in nine primary health care practices in Krakow. In every practice there was close cooperation with physicians and formal managers of the practice and two nurses and prevention managers.

The intervention curriculum was created with written materials concerning the basic information about diabetes, diabetes prevention, diet, a booklet with diet examples, and information about physical activity (available at www.image-project.eu).

The DE-PLAN Poland intervention was carried out by well-trained nurses, certified prevention managers, with knowledge on the subject and practical skills; special structured training on diabetes prevention and motivation techniques for the nurses was developed. A detailed description of design, education of prevention managers, and intervention strategy used in the DE-PLAN Poland project has been published elsewhere [21].

The study group consisted of patients of the primary health centers participating in the DE-PLAN project from 2006 to 2008. The inclusion criterion was a FINDRISC score >14 and exclusion criteria were known or OGTT-diagnosed diabetes [16]. In total, 175 people completed the intervention and the final examination. Intervention consisted of two parts: an intensive initial phase followed by an ongoing maintenance phase, and was based on reinforced behavior modification focusing on five lifestyle goals: weight loss, reduced intake of total and saturated fats, increased consumption of fruits, vegetables and fiber, and increased physical activity [21].

The intensive intervention phase, lasting 4 months, consisted of 10 group sessions (of 10–14 people) on lifestyle changes, diet, and physical activity education and was followed by a 6-month continuous phase, including six telephone motivation sessions and two motivation letters sent to the study participant.

Social support was emphasized by the group setting. Participants were also encouraged to involve their own social environment to participate in the lifestyle changes. A spouse or other family member could participate in the sessions. Study participants had also the opportunity to participate in physical activity sessions (aqua aerobic sessions and aerobic gym sessions) once or twice a week.

In all study participants, questionnaire (FINDRISC, basic and quality of life questionnaires) and biochemical tests (fasting and OGTT glucose (mmol/L), total, triglycerides, and high density lipoprotein (HDL) cholesterol (mmol/L) were examined before and 12 months after initiation of the intervention. Anthropometry of weight (kg), height (cm), BMI (kg/m^2), waist circumference (cm) and systolic and diastolic blood pressure (mmHg) were measured before and 12 months after initiation of the intervention and during selected group sessions as one of the motivation tools. Most of the study participants (78%) were women. They were slightly obese (mean BMI 31.5 kg/m^2 in men and 31.8 kg/m^2 in women) with abdominal fat distribution (waist circumference 106.1 cm in men and 96.7 cm in women). Men were heavier, had larger waist circumference, higher serum triglycerides, and lower HDL cholesterol than women ($P < 0.05$). IFG was more common in men than in women ($P < 0.05$).

Table 8.3 Poland: Changes in clinical outcome in baseline and after intervention.

	N	Baseline		After intervention		Change since baseline		Change (%)
		Mean	SD	Mean	SD	Mean	SD	
Fasting glucose (mmol/L)	175	5.28	0.75	5.39	0.65	0.11	0.72	−2.1
120 min OGTT glucose (mmol/L)	175	5.86	1.85	6.18	2.34	0.31	2.35	−5.4
Total cholesterol[a] (mmol/L)	175	5.56	1.00	5.33	0.98	0.23	1.16	4.2
HDL (mmol/L)	175	1.37	0.36	1.37	0.37	0.00	0.32	0.1
Triglicerydes (mmol/L)	175	1.76	1.18	1.63	0.80	0.13	1.14	7.2
WC (cm)[a]	175	98.77	11.81	95.51	11.99	3.26	6.11	3.3
Weight (kg)[a]	175	85.65	16.12	83.73	15.97	1.92	5.01	2.2
BMI (m/kg^2)[a]	175	31.76	5.01	31.07	4.98	0.69	1.90	2.2
SBP (mmHg)[a]	175	133.22	14.41	131.15	12.64	2.07	14.40	1.6
DBP (mmHg)[a]	175	82.98	8.52	81.02	8.96	1.96	9.01	2.4

BMI, body mass index; DBP, diastolic blood pressure; HDL, high density lipoprotein cholesterol; OGTT, oral glucose tolerance test; SBP, systolic blood pressure; WC, waist circumference.
[a]$P < 0.05$.

Table 8.3 shows changes in clinical outcome at baseline and after the intervention. At 12 months, participants' mean weight was reduced by 1.9 ± 5.0 kg (2.2%), BMI by 0.7 ± 1.9 kg/m^2 (2.2%) and waist circumference by 3.3 ± 6.1 cm (3.3%). A total of 24.6% of the study participants lost ≥5% of their initial body weight (mean loss 7.76 ± 5.70 kg), 40% lost ≤5% of initial body weight (mean loss 1.95 ± 1.22 kg), 14.7% did not change their weight, and 21.7% gained weight (mean weight gain 3.3 ± 2.8 kg). Mean fasting and post load plasma glucose did not change. Total cholesterol decreased by 4.2% (from 5.56 to 5.33 mmol/L, $P < 0.05$). Triglycerides and HDL cholesterol did not change. Systolic and diastolic blood pressure decreased from baseline 133.18 and 82.98 mmHg to 130.41 and 81.02 mmHg (by 1.6 and 2.4%, $P < 0.05$), respectively.

Of the study participants, 27 (15.4%) had IGT, 28 (16%) had IFG, and 131 (74.8%) were normoglycemic at baseline. After the intervention, IGT was present in 34 (19.4%), IFG in 20 (11.4%), and 125 (71.4%) were normoglycemic. Among patients with baseline IGT, 3 (11%) progressed to diabetes, and 11 (40%) reversed to NGT. Among patients with baseline IFG, 3 (10.7%) progressed to diabetes, and 10 (35.7%) reversed to NGT.

Table 8.4 Poland: Diet and physical activity at baseline and after intervention.

	Baseline (%)	After intervention (%)
I have increased consumption of vegetables, fruits during the past year*	24.0	51.4
I have changed saturated fat to unsaturated fat used during the past year*	29.1	61.7
I have decreased the amount of fat in my diet during the past year*	25.1	52.6
I think I exercise enough to maintain my physical condition or health*	9.7	20.0
I have increased physical activity during the past year[a]	7.4	25.7

[a]$P < 0.05$.

Out of the study participants with baseline normoglycemia, 3 (2.3%) progressed to diabetes, 15 (11.5%) progressed to IGT, and 7 (5.3%) progressed to IFG. The mean FINDRISC at baseline was 18.3 (SD = 2.84) indicating moderate to high diabetes risk (1 out of 3 persons would be expected to develop diabetes within the next 10 years) and decreased to 15.8 (3.77) after the intervention.

Significant improvements were also found in lifestyle risk factors (Table 8.4). At the end of the intervention, 51.4% of study participants increased fruit and vegetable consumption compared to baseline (24.0%, $P < 0.05$). Of study participants, 52.6 % and 61.7% diminished the total amount of fat in their diet and changed saturated fat into unsaturated (baseline 25.1% and 29.1%, respectively) ($P < 0.05$). Study participants increased physical activity during the intervention period (25.8% were physically active, compared with 7% at baseline, $P < 0.05$).

Discussion

The main conclusion drawn from both the Greek and Polish arms of the DE-PLAN project is that simple interventions for T2D prevention, based on lifestyle modification, are feasible in the community setting. Their effectiveness, however, seems to be lower when compared with clinical trials aiming to prevent T2D [6,7].

The Greek arm of the DE-PLAN focused, in part, at identifying factors related to the effectiveness of the recruitment procedure. It showed that considerable effort is needed to recruit people and to maintain them in a lifestyle intervention program for preventing T2D in the community. In Greece, recruitment from workplaces was more successful than from primary care centers. The distribution of risk calculation questionnaires in primary care resulted in the final enrolment of 118 individuals (1.8%), while in the occupational setting the rate was almost three times higher (4.8%) (Figure 8.1). This was mainly because of the higher rate of completed questionnaires (80% in occupational vs. 30% in primary care). This is a very high rate of return, as studies using mass mailings for recruitment typically enrol participants from 1–7% of letters sent [22].

The reasons for this discrepancy can only be speculated upon. When the FINDRISC questionnaires were distributed at the work sites during the "Day for diabetes prevention," people were informed personally about the project and had immediate and instant access to questions and answers. Thus, they were more easily persuaded to fill in the questionnairesthan in primary care settings, where leaflets were handed out to be filled in later at home. "Peer pressure" from colleagues and the fact that the intervention sessions would conveniently take place at their workplace may have motivated enrollment.

In both countries, the intervention program was of 1 year's duration and relied on group sessions, undertaken by dietitians (Greece) and specialized nurses (Poland). The main focus of both programs was the provision of information regarding a healthy diet. No special attention was given to the implementation of a structured exercise program and no behavioral change approach was attempted in Greece, whereas in Poland there was more intense counseling on physical activity and people could participate in 45 minutes of physical activity sessions once or twice a week (e.g., aqua aerobic sessions and/or aerobic gym sessions). A specialist experienced in physical activity changes in middle-aged people was used to train the nurses who participated in the project and gave physical activity sessions (aqua aerobic sessions and aerobic gym sessions). In fact, self-reported physical activity status improved after the intervention (Table 8.4).

Evidence from randomized controlled clinical trials has shown that lifestyle intervention, including dietary modification, weight loss, and physical activity, may reduce T2D incidence by up to 60% [5–10].

In order to determine the feasibility of the translation of the current research evidence into clinical settings within existing health care systems, several implementation programs worldwide have been performed. In the study by Laatikainen et al. [23], a structured group program with six 90-minutes sessions was delivered to 237 middle-aged individuals during an 8-month period by trained nurses in an Australian primary health care setting and resulted in weight and waist circumference reduction and improvement of cardiovascular risk factors. In addition, the GOAL lifestyle implementation trial demonstrated that lifestyle counseling may be effective and feasible in primary health care centers [24,25]. In that study, the intervention, with lifestyle change objectives drawn from the Diabetes Prevention Study (DPS), was delivered to 352 middle-aged people with increased diabetes risk (FINDRISC score = 16.2 ± 3.3), as six sessions at sociobehavioral group counseling by public health nurses over a period of 8 months. Statistically significant reduction achieved at 12 months of the intervention was maintained at 36 months in weight, BMI, and serum cholesterol [24,25]. Similar results were obtained in the Prevention of Diabetes Self-Management Programme (PREDIAS). In that program, 12 group sessions were delivered to 182 people with elevated diabetes risk, by diabetes educators or psychologists [26].

In the Greek and Polish arms of the DE-PLAN study, the effectiveness of the project regarding weight loss at 1 year (Greece 1.0%, Poland 2.2%) was clearly lower than the weight loss achieved in the intervention arm of the two landmark clinical trials (DPS 4.7%, Diabetes Prevention Program (DPP) 6.5%) [6,7]. Both community-based interventions were not as intense as the DPS study [6], where participants had seven individual counseling sessions with a nutritionist in the first year and also individual guidance and supervised individually tailored training sessions for increasing their physical activity levels. Certainly, the intensity of intervention in both the "real-world" projects was much weaker than in the DPP study [7], where each participant had 16 individual sessions – covering diet, exercise, and behavioral changes – with a case manager in the first 6 months of the study and monthly thereafter. This was probably the reason for the lower weight reduction success in our cohorts. Nevertheless, the intervention strategies used both in Greece and Poland were practical from a community standpoint and feasible for routine primary care. Identification of high-risk individuals through a questionnaire that requires minimal effort to fill in is also a great advantage from a community standpoint, because it can be easily implemented in routine primary care.

In both the Polish and Greek DE-PLAN studies the beneficial clinical and lifestyle changes were observed in all those who took part in the intervention; however, not surprisingly, changes were more pronounced in those who reached the goal of >5% of weight loss (24% of the individuals in the Polish and 15% in the Greek cohort [data not published]). In addition, in the Greek arm, effectiveness in weight loss was associated with closer adherence to the program, as reflected by the number of visits attended by the participants [19]. In both countries, a moderate regression of progression of dysglycemic status was observed. However, the lack of a control group and the relatively short duration of the interventions limits the possibility for solid conclusions to be drawn.

In summary, community-based lifestyle interventions aiming at T2D prevention, as implemented in the Greek and Polish arms of the DE-PLAN study, were feasible and showed promising results in terms of weight loss and improvement of cardiovascular risk factors. In Greece, recruitment from occupational settings was clearly superior to a primary care approach. In both countries, longer term data and larger cohorts are needed for solid conclusions regarding T2D prevention program design in the community.

References

1. King H, Aubert RE, Herman WH. Global burden of diabetes, 1995–2025. Prevalence, numerical estimates and projections. Diabetes Care 1998;21:1414–31.
2. Cowie CC, Rust KF, Ford ES, Eberhardt MS, Byrd-Holt DD, Li C, et al. Full accounting of diabetes and pre-diabetes in the US population in 1988–1994 and 2005–2006. Diabetes Care 2009;32:287–94.
3. Manuel DG, Schultz SE. Health-related quality of life and health-adjusted life expectancy of people with diabetes in Ontario, Canada, 1996–1997. Diabetes Care 2004;27(2):407–14.
4. Jönsson B. Revealing the cost of type II diabetes in Europe. Diabetologia 2002; 45:S5–S12.
5. Kahn SE. The relative contributions of insulin resistance and beta-cell dysfunction to the pathophysiology of type 2 diabetes. Diabetologia 2003;46:3–19.
6. Tuomilehto J, Lindstrom J, Eriksson JG, Valle TT, Hamalainen H, Ilanne-Parikka P, et al. Prevention of type 2 diabetes mellitus by changes in lifestyle among subjects with impaired glucose tolerance. N Engl J Med 2001;344:1343–50.
7. Knowler WC, Barrett-Connor E, Fowler SE, Hamman RF, Lachin JM, Walker EA, et al. Reduction in the incidence of type 2 diabetes with lifestyle intervention or metformin. N Engl J Med 2002;346:393–403.
8. Chiasson JL, Josse RG, Gomis R, Hanefeld M, Karasik A, Laakso M. Acarbose for prevention of type 2 diabetes mellitus: the stop-NIDDM randomised trial. Lancet 2002;359:2072–7.
9. DeFronzo RA, Tripathy D, Schwenke DC, Banerji MA, Bray GA, Buchanan TA, et al., for the ACT NOW Study. Pioglitazone for diabetes prevention in impaired glucose tolerance. N Engl J Med 2011;364:1104–15.

10. Paulweber B, Valensi P, Lindstrom J, Lalic NM, Greaves CJ, McKee M, et al. A European evidence-based guideline for the prevention of type 2 diabetes. Horm Metab Res 2010;42 (Suppl 1):S3–S36.

11. American Diabetes Association. Standards of medical care in diabetes – 2011. Diabetes Care 2011;34(Suppl 1):S11–61.

12. Ackermann RT, Finch EA, Brizendine E, Zhou H, Marrero DG. Translating the Diabetes Prevention Program into the community: the DEPLOY Pilot Study. Am J Prev Med 2008;35:357–63.

13. Costa B, Cabre JJ, Sagarra R, Sola-Morales O, Barrio F, Pinol JL, et al. for the DE-PLAN-CAT/PREDICE Research Group. Rationale and design of the PREDICE project: cost-effectiveness of type 2 diabetes prevention among high-risk Spanish individuals following lifestyle intervention in real-life primary care setting. BMC Public Health 2011;11:623.

14. Valensi P, Schwarz EH, Hall M, Felton AM, Maldonato A, Mathieu C. Pre-diabetes essential action: a European perspective. Diabetes Metab 2005;31:606–20.

15. Schwarz PE, Schwarz J, Schuppenies A, Bornstein SR, Schulze J. Development of a diabetes prevention management program for clinical practice. Public Health Rep 2007;122:258–63.

16. Schwarz PEH, Lindstrom J, Kissimova-Skarbeck K, Szybinski Z, Barengo NC, Peltonen M, et al. on behalf of the DE-PLAN project. The European perspective of type 2 diabetes prevention: Diabetes in Europe – Prevention using lifestyle, physical activity and nutritional intervention (DE-PLAN) project. Exp Clin Endocrinol Diabetes 2008;116:167–72.

17. Lindstrom J, Tuomilehto J. The Diabetes Risk Score: a practical tool to predict type 2 diabetes risk. Diabetes Care 2003;26:725–31.

18. World Medical Association Declaration of Helsinki. Recommendations guiding physicians in biomedical research involving human subjects. JAMA 1997;277:925–6.

19. Makrilakis K, Liatis S, Grammatikou S, Perrea D, Katsilambros N. Implementation and effectiveness of the first community lifestyle intervention program to prevent type 2 diabetes in Greece: The Deplan study. Diabet Med 2010;27:459–65.

20. Kontogianni MD, Liatis S, Grammatikou S, Perrea D, Katsilambros N, Makrilakis K. Changes in dietary habits and their association with metabolic markers after a non-intensive, community-based lifestyle intervention to prevent type 2 diabetes, in Greece: The DEPLAN study. Diabetes Res Clin Pract 2012;95:207–14.

21. Gilis-Januszewska A, Szybinski Z, Kissimova-Skarbek K, Piwońska-Solska B, Pach D, Topor-Madry R, et al. Prevention of type 2 diabetes by lifestyle intervention in primary health care setting in Poland: Diabetes in Europe Prevention using Lifestyle, Physical Activity and Nutritional intervention (DE-PLAN) Project. Br J Diabetes Vasc Dis 2011;11:198–203.

22. Cosgrove N, Borhani NO, Bailey G, Borhani P, Levin J, Hoffmeier M, et al. Mass mailing and staff experience in a total recruitment program for a clinical trial: the SHEP experience. Systolic Hypertension in the Elderly Program. Cooperative Research Group. Control Clin Trials 1999;20:133–48.

23. Laatikainen T, Dunbar JA, Chapman A, Kilkkinen A, Vartiainen E, Heistaro S, et al. Prevention of type 2 diabetes by lifestyle intervention in an Australian primary health care setting: Greater Green Triangle (GGT) Diabetes Prevention Project. BMC Public Health 2007;19:249.

24. Absetz P, Valve R, Oldenburg B, Heinonen H, Nissinen A, Fogelholm M, et al. Type 2 diabetes prevention in the "real world": one-year results of the GOAL Implementation Trial. Diabetes Care 2007;30:2465–70.

25. Absetz P, Oldenburg B, Hankonen N, Valve R, Heinonen H, Nissinen A, et al. Type 2 diabetes prevention in the real world: three-year results of the GOAL lifestyle implementation trial. Diabetes Care 2009;32:1418–20.

26. Kulzer B, Hermanns N, Gorges D, Schwarz P, Haak T. Prevention of diabetes self-management program (PREDIAS): effects on weight, metabolic risk factors, and behavioral outcomes. Diabetes Care 2009;32:1143–6.

CHAPTER 9

Quality management and outcome evaluation in diabetes prevention

Markku Peltonen[1] and Rüdiger Landgraf[2]

[1] Department of Chronic Disease Prevention, National Institute for Health and Welfare, Helsinki, Finland
[2] Department of Internal Medicine, Endocrinology and Diabetology, German Diabetes Foundation, Munich, Germany

Introduction

The increase in type 2 diabetes is a major public health problem worldwide [1]. In clinical trials, individuals at high risk for type 2 diabetes have significantly reduced their risk and delayed the onset of the disease by adopting a healthy, nutritionally balanced diet, increasing physical activity, and maintaining or reducing body weight [2–7]. Translating this evidence into improvements in public health necessitates the development and implementation of effective prevention strategies and programs [8].

The IMAGE project – Development and Implementation of a European Guideline and Training Standards for Diabetes Prevention – was initiated to unify and enhance the various prevention management concepts currently in circulation [9,10]. The main objectives were to develop evidence-based guidelines for the prevention of type 2 diabetes, a toolkit for practical implementation, a curriculum for prevention managers, and an e-learning portal for prevention activities. In addition, standards for quality management and outcome evaluation were produced for use in primary prevention [11,12].

Continuous quality control and evaluation of processes and outcomes are the key elements of a successful primary prevention program. Unified quality standards are required for systematic evaluation and reporting.

Prevention of Diabetes, First Edition. Edited by Peter Schwarz and Prasuna Reddy.
© 2013 John Wiley & Sons, Ltd. Published 2013 by John Wiley & Sons, Ltd.

Quality indicators for clinical diabetes care have been developed by several organizations and working groups. In contrast, quality management in diabetes prevention is underdeveloped. Currently, prevention programs frequently lack methods for structured follow-up and evaluation, and there are no standardized quality indicators available.

This chapter describes the quality and evaluation standards produced by the IMAGE project, and presents a set of quality and outcome evaluation indicators for diabetes prevention programs. The development of these indicators is described in detail in the original publications [11,12]. This chapter focuses on quality management in primary prevention, and is targeted at those responsible for diabetes prevention across the different levels of the health care system.

Quality in diabetes care

Quality in health care can be defined as "the degree to which health services for individuals and populations increase the likelihood of desired health outcomes and are consistent with current professional knowledge" [13]. Nonetheless, defining quality of health care is complex because of differing perspectives and approaches to defining, measuring, and improving it [14].

Evidence-based clinical guidelines are derived from the practice of evidence-based medicine. However, clinical guidelines do not in themselves guarantee quality of care. For example, a considerable portion of the diabetic population is not properly cared for despite the widespread availability of guidelines [15]. Indeed, it has been shown that clinical guidelines only improve clinical practice when their outcomes are evaluated [16].

Despite recommendations, quality indicators are not often incorporated into clinical guidelines [17]. Even the most esteemed international diabetes guidelines commonly lack systematic quality indicators [18–21]. However, the National Institute for Health and Clinical Excellence (NICE) [22] has published implementation tools including audit criteria and standards for guidelines to measure organizational practice against [23].

Several projects aimed at enhancing reporting of diabetes issues have been conducted at European level. The European Core Indicators for Diabetes Mellitus (EUCID) project (2006–2007) developed 27 indicators and demonstrated the feasibility of data collection in different EU countries and future Member States. The project aimed to promote planning for good diabetes health status and diabetes care organization in each country [24].

Many consortia have developed quality indicators specifically for clinical diabetes care. The Organisation for Economic Cooperation and Development (OECD) Quality Indicator Project has published a list of nine health system level quality indicators for diabetes care [25,26]. In the United States, the Diabetes Quality Improvement Project (DQIP) has developed and implemented a comprehensive and widely endorsed set of national measures for evaluation [27]. A working group including participants from 15 European Union/European Free Trade Area (EU/EFTA) countries has generated a set of 31 indicators for monitoring diabetes and its complications within EU/EFTA countries [28]. In several European countries efforts have been made to implement quality indicators in diabetes care. For example, in Germany the Saxon Diabetes Management Program has developed an integrated quality management system [29]. A Belgian study has produced a list of quality indicators for type 2 diabetes by evaluating 125 diabetes guidelines in five European countries [17]. One group in the Netherlands provided a set of quality indicators for the pharmacologic management of type 2 diabetes [30]. In the field of diabetes education, the International Diabetes Federation has published standards including quality indicators [31,32].

Quality in health promotion and primary prevention

In contrast to diabetes care, quality management and indicators in diabetes prevention are underdeveloped. Although many national organizations and consortia have developed guidelines for the prevention and management of obesity [33–35], only the NICE recommendations identify measurable indicators and include audit criteria, which help with their implementation [36].

The European Society of Cardiology guidelines on cardiovascular disease prevention in clinical practice [21] and on diabetic heart disease [19] similarly lack quality indicators. The American College of Cardiology Foundation/American Heart Association, in collaboration with other organizations, have recently published a curriculum [37] and performance measures for the primary prevention of cardiovascular disease in adults [38]. These provide tools for measuring the quality of care and help identify opportunities for improvement [38]. In Europe, a set of quality indicators for the prevention and management of cardiovascular disease in primary care was developed by experts representing nine countries [39].

Classification of quality and outcome indicators

The IMAGE quality indicators were designed to be applicable to the broadest possible population. They cover different prevention strategies and target actors at different levels of the health care system. The quality standards are divided into quality indicators and scientific outcome evaluation measurements. The quality indicators can be considered the minimum requirement for prevention activities, while the scientific outcome indicators enable evaluation.

Prevention strategy

The population-level prevention strategy aims to develop, improve, and implement primary prevention programs targeting the entire population. Successful population-level diabetes prevention requires the participation of numerous community stakeholders such as educational institutions, the food industry, media, urban planners, and nongovernmental organizations (NGOs).

The high-risk prevention strategy aims to identify high-risk individuals and support them with lifestyle changes required to reduce their risk for diabetes.

Effective screening for individuals at high risk for type 2 diabetes is essential for successful interventions. Different methods of screening include the use of risk questionnaires, opportunistic screening, and computer database searching. Long-lasting individual prevention is especially successful if behavioral changes are combined with setting adaptations.

Level of the health care operator

Depending on the level of the health care operator, different quality indicators are of interest. Macro-level indicators are important for representatives of the national-level health institutes and NGOs interested in diabetes prevention.

At the meso-level (i.e., the level of operative primary care) indicators are needed to assist diabetes prevention in health districts, health care centers, occupational health, the private sector, and local-level NGOs.

At the micro-level, indicators are required for personnel (physicians, nurses, dietitians, physiotherapists, specialized prevention managers) who carry out hands-on preventive work.

Table 9.1 Overview of classification of quality and outcome evaluation indicators.

Prevention strategy	
Population strategy	Activities aimed at promoting the health of entire population
High-risk intervention strategy	Identification of and interventions for at-risk individuals
Level of health care operator	
Macro level	National-level decision makers
Meso level	Operative primary health care level
Micro level	Individual-level prevention work
Quality criteria	
Structure indicators	Material and human resources, organizational structure
Process indicators	Activities undertaken to implement intervention
Quality and outcome indicators	
Outcome indicators	Effects of interventions and activities related to diabetes prevention
Scientific evaluation indicators	Outcome measures for evaluation purposes

Structure, process, and outcome model

The quality indicators presented here are classified according to the structure, process, and outcome (SPO) model [40,41]. Structure describes the material and human resources as well as organizational structure. These includes facilities, financing, and personnel. Process refers to activities undertaken to achieve objectives such as the giving and receiving of care and the implementation of interventions. Outcome describes the effect of care or interventions on the health status of a subject or population.

Table 9.1 presents an overview of classifications of the quality and outcome evaluation indicators developed by the IMAGE project.

Quality criteria and indicators

The SPO model provides the criteria for the quality indicators used for measuring diabetes prevention. Table 9.2 presents the structure and process quality criteria according to macro-, meso- and micro-levels of health care operator. The corresponding quality and outcome indicators to measure these criteria are given in Table 9.3.

Population-level prevention strategies

A successful population-level prevention strategy requires policies, legislation, and health monitoring systems supportive to obesity and diabetes

Table 9.2 Structure and process quality criteria for diabetes prevention by macro-, meso-, and micro-levels of health care operator.

Macro-level quality criteria

Policies and legislation support environment favoring diabetes prevention

A national diabetes prevention plan with specific prevention targets is available

National health monitoring systems provide sufficient information for the surveillance of diabetes

In all activities of diabetes prevention, ethnic minorities and low socioeconomic groups are considered

Policies and legislation take into account measures needed for prevention of obesity among children and adolescents

Meso-level quality criteria

Basic knowledge in population-level prevention of diabetes is part of the curricula of medical professionals working for health care provider

Health care providers are collaborating actively with other players active in health promotion

Different screening protocols have been evaluated at national level

Validated diabetes risk assessment tools are available to health care providers

Information technology systems supporting the implementation of screening are available at health care provider level

Defined clinical pathways exist for the health care provider to deal with individuals at risk for diabetes

Multidisciplinary approach for interventions is supported by the health care provider

High-risk prevention strategies are included in the education of the health care professionals

Medical record system supports interventions for chronic disease prevention

Micro-level quality criteria

Individual's risk factor profile is assessed

Individual's motivation for behavioral changes is discussed

Structure and content of the interventions have been defined at individual level

Individualized targets for interventions have been established

Plan for follow-up is defined

prevention. National diabetes prevention targets should include consideration of the special needs of ethnic minorities and underprivileged socioeconomic groups, because these groups have a higher than average incidence of type 2 diabetes. The prevention of obesity among children and adolescents should also be an objective. National health monitoring systems should provide sufficient information to enable effective surveillance.

At the health care provider level, diabetes prevention should be promoted and sufficient resources allocated to preventive work. Basic knowledge of population-level strategies for the prevention of diabetes should be included in the curricula of medical professionals. There should also be

Table 9.3 Quality and outcome indicators for a population-level prevention strategy and high-risk prevention strategies and corresponding levels of health care operator.

Population-level prevention strategy	Level
Proportion of population aware of diabetes and its risk factors	Macro
Prevalence of diabetes in the population	Macro
Percentage of the population physically inactive	Macro
Prevalence of overweight, obesity, and abdominal obesity in population	Macro
Percentage of population following national recommendations on nutrition	Macro
Percentage of health care costs allocated to prevention programs	Macro
Proportion of health care personnel per health care provider active in population-level primary prevention	Meso
Number of health promotion organizations active in population-level primary prevention	Meso
High-risk prevention strategy	**Level**
Proportion of the population screened by health care providers per year	Meso
Percentage of identified high-risk individuals directed to diagnostic procedures	Meso
Percentage of identified high-risk individuals directed to lifestyle interventions	Meso
Number of health care professionals at health care provider level qualified for interventions per 100 000 inhabitants	Meso
Percentage of remitted high-risk individuals participating in lifestyle interventions	Meso
Proportion of individuals dropping out of interventions	Meso
Proportion of high-risk individuals in interventions achieving clinically significant changes in risk factors at 1-year follow-up	Meso
Diabetes incidence rate among high-risk individuals in interventions	Meso
Proportion of planned intervention visits completed over 1 year	Micro
Weight change over 1 year	Micro
Change in waist circumference over 1 year	Micro
Change in glucose over 1 year	Micro
Change in the quality of nutrition over 1 year	Micro
Change in physical activity over 1 year	Micro

Source: from Pajunen et al. [12], with permission from Georg Thieme Verlag KG.

active collaboration between the different stakeholders in the health promotion field.

Decision makers can monitor and evaluate the quality and effectiveness of the selected population-level strategies by applying these quality indicators (Table 9.3).

High-risk prevention strategy

Screening protocols should be validated and evaluated at a national level before being implemented by the health care provider. They should contain a pathway for diagnostic procedures, as well as defined intervention strategies for different subgroups (e.g., age, minorities). The health care provider should promote validated diabetes risk assessment tools. Information technology systems should include screening tools.

Screening strategies at meso-level should incorporate clinical pathways for at-risk individuals. A multidisciplinary approach to interventions is recommended. Health care professionals should be educated in prevention strategies. Medical record systems should support interventions and chronic disease prevention in general.

At micro-level, the individual's risk factor profile should be assessed at the start of the intervention, and motivation for behavioral changes explored. The structure and content of interventions should be defined and individualized targets established. Individual follow-up should be planned and recorded.

Outcome evaluation indicators

Table 9.4 presents an example of the content included in micro-level data collection. These micro-level evaluation indicators provide outcome and performance measurements of diabetes prevention activities, and improve the quality of scientific evaluation and reporting. Local needs and circumstances are decisive for the final form of the data collection method adopted in different prevention programs.

Standardized and valid measurements are needed to obtain reliable and comparable results. Recommendations for standardized physical measurements (weight, height, waist circumference, blood pressure) are found in the Feasibility of European Health Examination Survey (FEHES) [42] and the World Health Organization (WHO) STEPS Manual [43].

The WHO Laboratory Diagnosis and Monitoring of Diabetes Mellitus 2002 paper [44] provides standards for glucose measurements including the oral glucose tolerance test (OGTT). All steps in the analytical process require attention [45]. Pre-analytical issues may seriously affect the quality of glucose assays. Glucose is lost through glycolysis and NaF has been used for decades to inhibit it. Additionally, ice slurry prevents pre-analytic glucose loss. However, new fluoride–citrate mixture tubes allow prolonged storage and transportation of samples and should be considered to assure a high quality measurement process [45,46].

The International Federation of Clinical Chemistry and Laboratory Medicine (IFCC) has published standards for HbA1c measurements [31,32].

Table 9.4 Micro-level outcome indicators and recommended contents of data collection to support, monitor and evaluate micro-level diabetes prevention.

	Core items	Additional items
1. Personal data	Personal identification	Marital status Education Ethnicity Employment status
2. Screening	Method used in screening Risk score type and result (if used) Reason for intervention	
3. Health and health behavior	Chronic diseases Regular medications Smoking:	Family history of diabetes and CVD
	Never/previously/currently	How often, products used
	Physical activity:	
	Type, frequency, intensity	Work-related, commuting, leisure
	Method used in measuring (e.g., interview, diary, recall, pedometers, accelerometers)	
	Nutrition:	
	Dietary pattern: consumption of vegetables, fruits, spreads and oil, bread and cereal (whole/refined grain), sweets, beverages, alcohol, etc.	Energy proportion (E%) of fat, saturated and trans fat, dietary fiber (g/day, g/1000 kcal), total energy, alcohol (g, E%), added sugar (g, E%)
	Method used in measuring (e.g., food diary, food frequency questionnaire or checklist)	
4. Clinical data (measured)	Body weight	2 hr OGTT glucose
	Body height	HbA1c
	Waist circumference	Lipids (total, LDL, HDL cholesterol and triglycerides)
	Fasting glucose	Additional measures (fasting, insulin, etc.)
	Systolic and diastolic blood pressure	
5. Content of the intervention	Type of intervention (group, individual, etc.) Frequency, duration and other details Targets for the intervention:	
	Weight, diet, smoking, physical activity	
	Reinforcement	
6. Success of the intervention	Adherence (proportion of planned intervention visits completed) Changes in: health and health behavior and clinical data	Diabetes Treatment Satisfaction Questionnaire Health-related quality of life
7. Maintenance	Plans how to sustain possible lifestyle changes after intervention	

CVD, cardiovascular disease; HDL, high density lipoprotein; LDL, low density lipoprotein; OGTT, oral glucose tolerance test

Source: from Pajunen et al. [12], with permission from Georg Thieme Verlag KG.

Major differences exist between commercially available insulin assays. An IFCC Standardization of Insulin Assays working group has been established with the American Diabetes Association and is currently developing a candidate reference method for insulin analysis.

FEHES and the US Centers for Disease Control and Prevention (CDC) [47], which has a certification program for lipid measurements, provide recommendations on blood sampling.

Dietary pattern and composition can be evaluated using food diaries, food frequency questionnaires, and checklists. The method adopted depends upon cultural background, available resources, and the level of cooperation of high-risk persons. Culturally specific food composition databases are mandatory for accurate calculation of nutrient intakes. The quality of diet and dietary changes can be assessed by frequency of consumption of recommended (e.g., vegetables, fruit, whole grains) and non-recommended (e.g., soft drinks, pastries) food items.

Physical activity can be accurately measured using pedometers and accelerometers. Self-reported data can be collected via interviews, diaries, and recalls. Assessment should include type (e.g., walking, swimming), frequency (number of sessions), duration, and intensity (level of physical effort) of physical activity. Using these four components, relative energy expenditure can be estimated in metabolic equivalents (METS) [48].

The European Health Interview Survey (EHIS) includes standardized questions on use of medications [49]. Health economic evaluation and cost issues are considered in the IMAGE Scientific Guidelines [9]. Quality of life should be measured using standardized instruments and possible translations should be certified. Treatment satisfaction can be measured using the Diabetes Treatment Satisfaction Questionnaire (DTSQ) [50].

Discussion

The IMAGE evidence-based guideline [9] and practical guide for prevention [10] present a set of quality and outcome indicators for diabetes prevention. These indicators are therefore closely linked to the guideline standards, and can be used as performance measurements against both evidence-based and practical guidelines for diabetes prevention. The quality indicators provide decision makers, health care providers, and health care personnel with the tools to monitor, evaluate, and improve the quality of diabetes prevention. The implementation of quality management criteria may need adaptation to local circumstances depending on national and local legislation.

Both population-level and high-risk prevention strategies were considered when developing the indicators. The quality indicators represent different dimensions of preventive work: population-level prevention, screening for high risk and high-risk prevention. To promote usability the indicators were generated to be applicable to the broadest possible population: the definition of high-risk population covers all subjects at risk for type 2 diabetes irrespective of the screening method used, and the indicators apply to all adult age groups and to both sexes.

Methods of measuring and evaluating performance in health care are under constant development. In general, quality indicators are evidence-based measures that assess a particular health care structure, process or outcome [41]. They aim to provide a quantitative base for organizations, planners, and service providers to improve processes and care [51]. To measure quality reliably requires that criteria and standards are based on a scientifically validated fund of knowledge [52], or at least on the most authoritative opinion in a particular subject area [41]. A valid indicator must be reproducible and consistent. Validity is the degree to which an indicator measures its intended target (i.e., validity occurs when the result of a measurement corresponds to the state of the phenomenon being measured) [51]. Reliability is the extent to which an indicator measurement is reproducible. Reliability ensures that indicators can be used to make comparisons among or within groups over time [51].

The implementation of quality and outcome indicators needs adaptation to local circumstances. In Germany, the Coordination and Quality in Prevention (KoQuaP; www.koquap.de) system conforms to data protection laws while allowing all relevant data for measuring prevention to be submitted online. Management and evaluation of pseudonymized data can be performed by persons providing the interventions.

The quality indicators presented in this chapter are intended to be used in prospective settings but may be applicable for retrospective analysis if the quality of data collection enables this. They comprise the minimum level of quality standards necessary when developing and implementing diabetes prevention activities. Individuals and organizations using these measures are encouraged to involve a scientific evaluation perspective in preventive work by using the additional outcome evaluation indicators.

In conclusion, parallel with the development of the IMAGE guidelines for the prevention of type 2 diabetes, a quality management system with quality and outcome evaluation indicators and audit tools has been developed. The indicators are presented for different levels of the health care system. They can be used for internal quality control and for external comparison between operators, and they enable comparison between different prevention approaches. These quality standards complement the IMAGE guidelines and provide a tool for improving the quality of diabetes prevention.

Acknowledgment

This work is based on the products developed by the IMAGE European study group; please see www.image-project.eu.

References

1. Whiting DR, Guariguata L, Weil C, Shaw J. IDF Diabetes Atlas: Global estimates of the prevalence of diabetes for 2011 and 2030. Diabetes Res Clin Pract 2011; 94:311–21.
2. Tuomilehto J, Lindstrom J, Eriksson JG, Valle TT, Hamalainen H, Ilanne-Parikka P, et al. Prevention of type 2 diabetes mellitus by changes in lifestyle among subjects with impaired glucose tolerance. N Engl J Med 2001;344(18):1343–50.
3. Lindstrom J, Ilanne-Parikka P, Peltonen M, Aunola S, Eriksson JG, Hemio K, et al. Sustained reduction in the incidence of type 2 diabetes by lifestyle intervention: follow-up of the Finnish Diabetes Prevention Study. Lancet 2006;368(9548): 1673–9.
4. Knowler WC, Barrett-Connor E, Fowler SE, Hamman RF, Lachin JM, Walker EA, et al. Reduction in the incidence of type 2 diabetes with lifestyle intervention or metformin. N Engl J Med 2002;346(6):393–403.
5. Li G, Zhang P, Wang J, Gregg EW, Yang W, Gong Q, et al. The long-term effect of lifestyle interventions to prevent diabetes in the China Da Qing Diabetes Prevention Study: a 20-year follow-up study. Lancet 2008;371(9626):1783–9.
6. Ramachandran A, Snehalatha C, Mary S, Mukesh B, Bhaskar AD, Vijay V. The Indian Diabetes Prevention Programme shows that lifestyle modification and metformin prevent type 2 diabetes in Asian Indian subjects with impaired glucose tolerance (IDPP-1). Diabetologia 2006;49(2):289–97.
7. Kosaka K, Noda M, Kuzuya T. Prevention of type 2 diabetes by lifestyle intervention: a Japanese trial in IGT males. Diabetes Res Clin Pract 2005;67(2):152–62.
8. Schwarz PE, Schwarz J, Schuppenies A, Bornstein SR, Schulze J. Development of a diabetes prevention management program for clinical practice. Public Health Rep 2007;122(2):258–63.
9. Paulweber B, Valensi P, Lindstrom J, Lalic NM, Greaves CJ, McKee M, et al. A European evidence-based guideline for the prevention of type 2 diabetes. Horm Metab Res. 2010;42(Suppl 1):S3–36.

10. Lindstrom J, Neumann A, Sheppard KE, Gilis-Januszewska A, Greaves CJ, Handke U, et al. Take action to prevent diabetes: the IMAGE toolkit for the prevention of type 2 diabetes in Europe. Horm Metab Res 2010;42(Suppl 1):S37–55.

11. Pajunen P, Landgraf R, Muyelle F, Neumann A, Lindström J, Schwarz PE, et al. Quality and Outcome Indicators for Prevention of Type 2 Diabetes In Europe: IMAGE. Helsinki: THL, 2010.

12. Pajunen P, Landgraf R, Muylle F, Neumann A, Lindstrom J, Schwarz PE, et al. Quality indicators for the prevention of type 2 diabetes in Europe: IMAGE. Horm Metab Res. 2010;42(Suppl 1):S56–63.

13. Lohr K. Medicare: A Strategy for Quality Assurance, Vols 1 and 2. Washington, DC: National Academy Press; 1990.

14. Blumenthal D. Part 1: Quality of care: what is it? N Engl J Med 1996;335(12):891–4.

15. Gnavi R, Picariello R, Karaghiosoff L, Costa G, Giorda C. Determinants of quality in diabetes care process: the population-based Torino Study. Diabetes Care 2009; 32:1986–92.

16. Grimshaw JM, Russell IT. Effect of clinical guidelines on medical practice: a systematic review of rigorous evaluations. Lancet 1993;342(8883):1317–22.

17. Wens J, Dirven K, Mathieu C, Paulus D, Van Royen P. Quality indicators for type-2 diabetes care in practice guidelines: an example from six European countries. Prim Care Diabetes 2007;1(1):17–23.

18. IDF Clinical Guidelines Task Force. Global guideline for type 2 diabetes: recommendations for standard, comprehensive, and minimal care. Diabet Med 2006;23(6): 579–93.

19. Ryden L, Standl E, Bartnik M, Van den Berghe G, Betteridge J, de Boer MJ, et al. Guidelines on diabetes, pre-diabetes, and cardiovascular diseases: executive summary. The Task Force on Diabetes and Cardiovascular Diseases of the European Society of Cardiology (ESC) and of the European Association for the Study of Diabetes (EASD). Eur Heart J 2007;28(1):88–136.

20. Buse JB, Ginsberg HN, Bakris GL, Clark NG, Costa F, Eckel R, et al. Primary prevention of cardiovascular diseases in people with diabetes mellitus: a scientific statement from the American Heart Association and the American Diabetes Association. Circulation 2007;115(1):114–26.

21. Graham I, Atar D, Borch-Johnsen K, Boysen G, Burell G, Cifkova R, et al. European guidelines on cardiovascular disease prevention in clinical practice: full text. Fourth Joint Task Force of the European Society of Cardiology and other societies on cardiovascular disease prevention in clinical practice (constituted by representatives of nine societies and by invited experts). Eur J Cardiovasc Prev Rehabil 2007;14(Suppl 2):S1–113.

22. National Institute for Health and Clinical Excellence (NICE). Type 2 diabetes national clinical guideline for management in primary and secondary care (update). 2008.

23. National Institute for Health and Clinical Excellence (NICE). Audit support. Type 2 diabetes: clinical criteria. 2008. Available from: http://guidance.nice.org.uk/CG66/AuditSupport/clinical (accessed 20 March 2013).

24. European Core Indicators for Diabetes Mellitus (EUCID). Final report European Core Indicators in Diabetes project. 2008. Available from: http://ec.europa.eu/health/ph_projects/2005/action1/docs/action1_2005_frep_11_en.pdf (accessed 6 March 2013).

25. Greenfield S, Nicolucci A, Mattke S. Selecting indicators for the quality of diabetes care at the health system level in OECD countiries. OECD health technical papers. 2004.

26. Nicolucci A, Greenfield S, Mattke S. Selecting indicators for the quality of diabetes care at the health systems level in OECD countries. Int J Qual Health Care 2006;18(Suppl 1):26–30.

27. Fleming BB, Greenfield S, Engelgau MM, Pogach LM, Clauser SB, Parrott MA. The Diabetes Quality Improvement Project: moving science into health policy to gain an edge on the diabetes epidemic. Diabetes Care 2001;24(10):1815–20.

28. de Beaufort CE, Reunanen A, Raleigh V, Storms F, Kleinebreil L, Gallego R, et al. European Union diabetes indicators: fact or fiction? Eur J Public Health 2003;13(3 Suppl):51–4.

29. Rothe U, Muller G, Schwarz PE, Seifert M, Kunath H, Koch R, et al. Evaluation of a diabetes management system based on practice guidelines, integrated care, and continuous quality management in a Federal State of Germany: a population-based approach to health care research. Diabetes Care 2008;31(5):863–8.

30. Martirosyan L, Braspenning J, Denig P, de Grauw WJ, Bouma M, Storms F, et al. Prescribing quality indicators of type 2 diabetes mellitus ambulatory care. Qual Saf Health Care 2008;17(5):318–23.

31. American Diabetes Association; European Association for the Study of Diabetes; International Federation of Clinical Chemistry and Laboratory Medicine; International Diabetes Federation. Consensus statement on the worldwide standardisation of the HbA1c measurement. Diabetologia 2007;50(10):2042–3.

32. Implementation of standardization of HbA1c measurement. Summary of the meeting with manufacturers held in Milan, Italy, December 12, 2007. Clin Chem Lab Med 2008;46(4):573–4.

33. World Health Organization (WHO). Obesity: preventing and managing the global epidemic. Report of a WHO consultation on obesity. WHO Technical Report Series 2000.

34. Tsigos C, Hainer V, Basdevant A, Finer N, Fried M, Mathus-Vliegen E, et al. Management of obesity in adults: European clinical practice guidelines. Obes Facts 2008; 1:106–16.

35. Klein S, Sheard NF, Pi-Sunyer X, Daly A, Wylie-Rosett J, Kulkarni K, et al. Weight management through lifestyle modification for the prevention and management of type 2 diabetes: rationale and strategies: a statement of the American Diabetes Association, the North American Association for the Study of Obesity, and the American Society for Clinical Nutrition. Diabetes Care 2004;27(8):2067–73.

36. National Institute for Health and Clinical Excellence (NICE). Audit criteria. Obesity: Guidance on the prevention, identification, assessment and management of overweight and obesity in adults and children. 2006: Available from: http://guidance.nice.org.uk/CG43/AuditSupport (accessed 20 March 2013).

37. Bairey Merz CN, Alberts MJ, Balady GJ, Ballantyne CM, Berra K, Black HR, et al. ACCF/AHA/ACP 2009 competence and training statement: a curriculum on prevention of cardiovascular disease. Circulation 2009;120(13):e100–26.

38. Redberg RF, Benjamin EJ, Bittner V, Braun LT, Goff DC Jr, Havas S, et al. ACCF/AHA 2009 performance measures for primary prevention of cardiovascular disease in adults. Circulation 2009;120(13):1296–336.

39. Campbell SM, Ludt S, Van Lieshout J, Boffin N, Wensing M, Petek D, et al. Quality indicators for the prevention and management of cardiovascular disease in primary care in nine European countries. Eur J Cardiovasc Prev Rehabil 2008;15(5):509–15.

40. Donabedian A. Evaluating the quality of medical care. Milbank Mem Fund Q. 1966;44(3 Suppl):166–206.

41. Donabedian A. The quality of care. How can it be assessed? JAMA 1988;260(12): 1743–8.

42. Tolonen H, Koponen P, Aromaa A, Conti S, Graff-Iversen S, Grotvedt L, et al. for the feasibility of a European Health Examination Survey (FEHES) Project. Recommendations for the Health Examination Surveys in Europe. 2008. Available from: http://urn.fi/URN:ISBN:978-951-740-838-7 (accessed 20 March 2013).

43. World Health Organization (WHO). STEPwise approach to surveillance (STEPS). Part 3: Training and Practical Guides 3-3-14. Section 3: Guide to Physical Measurements (Step 2) 2008 [updated 2008; cited 2009 21 October]; Available from: http://www.who.int/chp/steps/Part3_Section3.pdf (accessed 6 March 2013).

44. World Health Organization (WHO). Laboratory Diagnosis and Monitoring of Diabetes Mellitus 2002. 2002 [updated 2002; cited 2009 21 October]; Available from: http://whqlibdoc.who.int/hq/2002/9241590483.pdf (accessed 6 March 2013).

45. Bruns DE, Knowler WC. Stabilization of glucose in blood samples: why it matters. Clin Chem 2009;55(5):850–2.

46. Gambino R, Piscitelli J, Ackattupathil TA, Theriault JL, Andrin RD, Sanfilippo ML, et al. Acidification of blood is superior to sodium fluoride alone as an inhibitor of glycolysis. Clin Chem 2009;55(5):1019–21.

47. Centers for Disease Control and Prevention (CDC). The Cholesterol Reference Method Laboratory Network (CRMLN). 2009. Available from: http://www.cdc.gov/labstandards/crmln.html (accessed 6 March 2013).

48. Kriska A, Caspersen C. Introduction to a collection of physical activity questionnaires. Med Sci Sports Exerc 1997;29(6 Suppl):S5–9.

49. European Health Interview Survey (EHIS). EHIS Questionnaire 2006. Available from: http://ec.europa.eu/health/ph_information/implement/wp/systems/docs/ev_20070315_ehis_en.pdf (accessed 6 March 2013).

50. Bradley C. The Diabetes Treatment Satisfaction Questionnaire (DTSQ). In: Bradley C, editor. Handbook of Psychology and Diabetes: a guide to psychological measurement in diabetes research and practice. Switzerland: Harwood Academic Publishers; 1994. pp. 111–32.

51. Mainz J. Defining and classifying clinical indicators for quality improvement. Int J Qual Health Care 2003;15(6):523–30.

52. Sackett D, Straus S, Richardson W. Evidence-Based Medicine: How to Practice and Teach EBM, 2nd edn. London: Churchill Livingstone; 2000.

CHAPTER 10

Training of prevention managers

Peter Kronsbein
Niederrhein University of Applied Sciences, Faculty of Nutrition, Food, and Hospitality Sciences, Mönchengladbach, Germany

Counseling persons at risk for type 2 diabetes mellitus is an ambitious challenge. We have learned from various studies that lifestyle changes can prevent or delay the manifestation of the disease (see Chapter 1) but sustained behavior change is an enormous effort and persons at risk need well-trained experienced people to support their intentions to establish and maintain a modified lifestyle. Usually, these lifestyle changes aim at modest weight loss and an increase in physical activity.

In the field of manifest diabetes mellitus, the education and empowerment of patients was already propagated by Joslin [1,2] as an integral part of treatment since the early years of insulin therapy. However, it took more than half a century (from 1923 till the late 1970s) for the beneficial effects of patient self-management to be widely accepted – owing to numerous studies on the results of diabetes treatment and teaching programs. In order to optimize patients' disease-related skills, knowledge, decisions, attitudes, and actions, structured patient education and treatment programs are implemented in many health care systems for type 1 and 2 diabetes.

In the context of these treatment activities, the diabetes educator was incorporated into the therapeutical team and this profession has now been established for many decades. The journal *The Diabetes Educator,* first published in 1975, has a considerable history of nearly 40 years. In many countries a specially structured training course and certification for diabetes educators have been established.

With respect to diabetes prevention the situation is completely different. The level of appreciation and dissemination of structured education and empowerment is to a certain extent some decades behind schedule. The beneficial effects of lifestyle intervention programs on the incidence of type 2 diabetes [3] have been published and the next aim is to implement certified diabetes prevention programs into national health care systems.

Together with these intentions and activities the role of the prevention manager in the field of type 2 diabetes (PM[T2Dm]) was recently established. PM training courses have been developed mostly based upon a specially structured training curriculum and defined certification regulations. In the IMAGE project (2007–2010), project partners from 15 European countries worked together to develop guidelines on diabetes prevention as well as a curriculum for the training of PM[T2Dm]. This curriculum was tested for practicability and acceptance in a pilot study in several project partner countries [4,5]. Some examples from the IMAGE curriculum for PM[T2Dm] are shown in this chapter.

Curriculum development for the training of prevention managers in the field of type 2 diabetes prevention

Within diabetes therapy, the majority of train-the-trainer programs for diabetes educators are "structured." This is also valid for treatment and teaching programs for people with diabetes. The format of a structured intervention makes sense as well for training and empowerment in the field of diabetes prevention.

The structured way to carry out a train-the-trainer program is first to define and then to follow a basic curriculum. Such a curriculum contains at least three important parts:

1. Description of the basic organizational conditions;
2. Definition of major learning objectives and specific learning goals, teaching methods, and didactical material; and
3. Definition of how to control the achievement of the learning objectives.

Best aspects of a curriculum concept are as follow:

- Training takes into account the existing or defined (pre-) conditions;
- During the planning phase, learning objectives as well as methods and didactical material are well defined; and
- The execution of the training, the duration of the training modules, and the examination regulations follow a standardized path which prevents discrepancies between different lecturers and places.

Description of basic organizational conditions

The development of a structured method for training and intervention needs to consider the political and organizational conditions of the country. These underlying regulations influence: (i) the structure of a lifestyle change intervention for the intended target group, and (ii) the train-the-trainer program for prevention managers.

As a precondition for the development of a curriculum for the training of prevention managers, various basic questions have to be answered:

- What are the conditions and regulations of the health care system for the implementation of diabetes prevention interventions?
- What are the tasks of the prevention managers in each country?
- What are the necessary entrance qualifications to enter PM training?
- What should the duration of PM training be?
- What is the didactical structure of the training modules?
- Will e-learning components be integrated into the training concept?

What are the conditions and regulations of the health care system for the implementation of diabetes prevention interventions?

There are various possible settings for the establishment of diabetes prevention interventions, such as private, public, or workplace settings. Also, strong community partners may implement and disseminate lifestyle interventions.

In Germany, for example, the majority of the population are members of a compulsory health insurance. At the primary health care level patients are attended by general practitioners and specialists in *private* practice and in clinics. Health care costs are covered by health insurance companies, which receive a monthly obligatory percentage of the salary of the insured. However, people at risk have to pay the fees for prevention interventions by themselves. Private nutritionists/dietitians or specialized physicians and physiotherapists/sports scientists offer group prevention programs according to a guideline published by health insurance companies [6]. If the required conditions are met (e.g., the qualification of the specialist, the content and number of sessions, the frequency of participation), a certain portion of lifestyle intervention costs (up to 150 €/year) is refunded by the health insurance company to the participant in the prevention program. The rules for partial refund were not designed especially for the prevention of diabetes, but could be applied to this.

Despite this partial refund of prevention costs, such a system is far from perfect because it excludes people of low economic status from diabetes prevention programs. These people cannot afford the initial expenses, even if they might be refunded later. So this group of society, which may benefit most from prevention interventions (because of its high prevalence of obesity and sedentarism), actually has little access to services offered privately.

The professionals who are most suitable to be trained as prevention managers are nutritionists/dietitians and experts in physical activity according to the regulations for actors in primary prevention issued by the German health insurance companies.

In most countries the health care services are *public* and primary health care is anchored in primary care units. Health costs are covered by state-funded national health services. Traditionally, primary prevention does not belong to the tasks of the primary health care team. Although millions of citizens may benefit from access to structured diabetes prevention interventions, there is a scarcity of public health care models for nationwide dissemination of screening and preventative interventions as a regular part of the national health care system. As long as primary prevention is not officially declared as a part of the services at health care units, prevention will only be carried out in places with a dedicated head of the unit and motivated personnel – and as something in addition to daily obligations. The most suitable professionals in this setting are highly motivated members of the health care team, such as dietitians/nutritionists, physiotherapists/sports scientists, nurses, health trainers, health care assistants, and health psychologists.

The *workplace* is a setting that has strong potential for health promotion and disease prevention. Finland, for example, has a long history of occupational health centers and the necessary experience and infrastructure to offer diabetes prevention programs. In other countries, middle-sized and large companies have occupational medical departments and health centers for their employees, providing an excellent basis for diabetes prevention interventions. For example, the BASF company in Ludwigshafen, Germany, each year has a special health topic. In 2006 it was Diabetes and diabetes prevention [7]. Small companies have the opportunity to support lifestyle change intentions of their employees by hiring private dietitians, PA experts, or health trainers for in-house programs or by paying the course fees for offsite activities.

Regrettably, the concept that the workplace is an important area for health campaigns is not yet widely accepted [8]. Health promotion is underrepresented especially in small and medium-sized companies work-places. There are several reasons for this. On the one hand, there is a lack of knowledge and awareness of the possibilities (e.g., refunding and organizational support from health insurance companies). On the other hand, there is no manpower to organize structured prevention activities which have to follow certain regulations. Another factor is that most of the persons in charge (executive directors) see no added value to support prevention activities within the company. Results on the financial return of respective activities are contradictory, and conclusions about the overall profitability cannot be made, because additional types of benefits – not yet represented in existing calculation models – have to be considered [9].

Additional obstacles from the employees' point of view in this setting are the fear of a lack of discretion in respect to individual health details and of a possible stigmatization of those employees who are – within a screening for prediabetes – detected as at "high risk" and who are subsequently asked to attend a respective in-house intervention program.

The delivery of diabetes prevention programs in the *community* by strong community partners is another approach. National, regional, and community-based associations, societies, and parishes can serve as a suitable basis for such health activities. For example, in the United States the Diabetes Prevention Program (DPP) was successfully translated into the community in partnership with the YMCA [10]. In the case of the DPP–YMCA partnership "wellness instructors" were specially trained to deliver the adapted community version of the DPP [11].

For a successful development of a training curriculum it is crucial to be aware of the local political and organizational situation. If local prerequisites are not respected, the training course may graduate well educated prevention managers who finally are not able to carry out lifestyle change interventions for people at risk because political, infrastructural, and/or monetary aspects inhibit its implementation.

What are the tasks of the prevention managers in the respective country?

Depending on the health care system, on the grade of infrastructural implementation of diabetes prevention, on the number of supporting partners in and outside the health care team, the tasks of the PM^{T2Dm} range from pure education activities for people at risk to management tasks in order to start a lifestyle change intervention program and implement it into the daily routine of the respective institution.

The management part includes:

- The organization of the program (including number and duration of teaching units, content of these units, teaching material, time-line/ dates, places, co-workers, costs for the participants, reimbursement, evaluation management);
- The motivation and recruitment of participants (target group, people at risk); and
- Interorganizational and intraorganizational networking.

Furthermore, the PM^{T2Dm} has a responsibility to *teach, counsel, and train* persons at risk on prevention related aspects of nutrition and physical activity. Recommended methods of behavior change and motivation are applied [4].

To be conscious of the tasks of the PM is important for the development of a curriculum because the tasks can be extensive. The less established prevention structures are, the more extensive the management tasks will be.

What are the necessary entrance qualifications to enter PM training?

Those who are expected to offer and carry out lifestyle intervention programs for people at risk for type 2 diabetes should be experienced in patient or client education. They should have the necessary knowledge and skills in the relevant intervention areas (nutrition, physical activities), and should be motivated and available in the respective health care system.

On the basis of these conditions and the tasks of the PM, the entrance qualifications for the training course of European prevention managers were defined in the IMAGE project as follows:

Available personnel within the respective national health care system, who are – according to the situation of the respective country – most appropriate, recognized and best educated

- to fulfil the management tasks (program organisation, recruitment of participants/ persons at risk, networking, cooperation with co-workers, and evaluation) as well as
- to teach, counsel, and train the two basis components of lifestyle change based on recommended methods of behaviour change and motivation: nutrition and physical activity.

In some countries the prevention manager will establish a multidisciplinary *diabetes prevention team*, aiming at the expertise integration of the respective prevention areas [4].

Consequently, the careful selection of professionals to be trained (available, most appropriate, recognized, and best educated within the national system) defines the target group for attending the PM training course.

What should the duration of PM training be?

The better the basic qualifications of the PM trainees, the shorter the training need be. If the PM course is offered as a study program for high school graduates it would need to be several years in duration because the basic principles of primary prevention and its intervention areas have to be taught. If the course is offered to experienced health care professionals with a suitable basic qualification, the PM training can be completed within a few days, focusing specifically on diabetes prevention. Specific aspects of physical activity and nutrition including the relevant behavioral change methods, evaluation management, and program organization would be taught. The latter two aspects only need covering briefly in the course if the whole field of prevention program organization, recruitment of persons at risk, networking, and evaluation (management tasks) is assumed by an established overseeing department.

Taking the defined tasks and entrance qualifications described above as a basis, the European IMAGE project for PM training proposed a program with eight modules (Table 10.1): seven face-to-face training units (Modules 1–6 and 8) of one training day per unit and a longitudinal project report (Module 7).

It was proposed that the overall timespan of the PM training course covers about 6 months (e.g., one training unit every 3–4 weeks). Immediately after the first face-to-face training day, the PM^{T2Dm} trainees should start to plan and organize a local prevention program [4]. At the next PM training days – with 4-week intervals – participants have the opportunity to discuss their experiences and problems with their colleagues and lecturers. This time structure may help to overcome difficulties of the local implementation process (Figure 10.1).

Of course, local circumstances and conditions will influence the time structure. So there might be other schemes, like linking together two

Table 10.1 Structure and core contents of the IMAGE PM^{T2Dm} training course.

Module 1	Problem, evidence, and tasks
Module 2	Diabetes prevention course organization, recruitment of participants (people at risk), networking, evaluation management
Modules 3 and 5	Behavior change and motivation
Module 4	Specific aspects of physical activity in diabetes prevention
Module 6	Specific aspects of nutrition in diabetes prevention
Module 7	Elaboration of an individual longitudinal project report
Module 8	Presentation and discussion of the project reports

A Curriculum for the Training of Prevention Managers (PM)

Time structure of PM training and local implementation of a prevention program

PM Training:

7 modules (M): **face-to-face**; **1 day each**;
            proposed interval: every 3–4 weeks

M1   M2   M3   M4   M5   M6   ,M8

plu‹ Module M7: individual **project report**

Time   ‹e   3 months   6 months   9 months   1 year   years

Organization of a local prevention program for
persons at risk

                    Start of the first **prevention course,**
                    sustained implementation of the program

Figure 10.1 Proposal for the time structure of a 7-day training program for diabetes prevention managers.

modules at two consecutive days or even blocking six modules in one intense training week. However, if the timespan of the whole PM training course (from the first to the last module) is very short, there will be little or no time to discuss the different local experiences of the implementation process of diabetes prevention programs. In any case, the presentation of the individual project reports (Module 8) is recommended to be scheduled about 6 months after the start of the PM training course in order to be able to assess local target achievement and success.

What is the didactical structure of the training modules?

The module-related part of the PM training course is by means of pre-course assignments and by lectures. In addition, the lectures consolidate the newly acquired knowledge and make it applicable in PM's daily activities. Working group activities on module-related key questions help to achieve this. Outside the face-to-face modules, post-module assignments complement the training.

Didactical structure and components of the training modules:
1. Pre-module assignments.
2. Face-to-face unit with:
   • Lectures; and
   • Working group activities on key questions.
3. Post-module assignments.

Within the face-to-face units, the lecture time (imparting facts and knowledge) should be limited so that there is time to work on group activities. Within working groups (e.g., in pairs) the PM trainees can be asked to work on key questions related to the learning unit and present their results to the plenary group. Such key questions should be designed by the lecturer of the module.

Examples of key questions for the first PM training module (problem, evidence, and tasks):

- Explain the study design – including the intervention goals – of the Finnish Diabetes Prevention Study to a colleague of your local health care team;
- Explain the results of the Finnish Diabetes Prevention Study to a journalist;
- Explain what "impaired glucose tolerance" means to a patient or person at risk;
- Explain the characteristics of an "oral glucose tolerance test."

After a given time (e.g., 30 minutes), the working group members are asked to present their results; certain aspects may be visualized (e.g., flip-chart, board). If the lecturer focuses on the communication with target groups, role-play is appropriate.

The time limit of presentation of the working group results (e.g., 10 minutes) should be respected and controlled in order to stay within the time schedule of the training module.

Will e-learning components be integrated into the training concept?

An e-learning platform can be helpful and supportive to the successful performance of a PM training course. Useful components are associated pre-module and post-module assignments, time schedules, protocols, guidelines, and drafts, as well as an online communication forum for the lecturers and trainees of the PM^{T2Dm} training course (for further details see Chapter 12).

Definition of learning objectives, methods, and materials

The description and definition of basic organizational aspects, as shown above, are a prerequisite for the development of the structure of the teaching and training process which recruits suitable trainees and delivers trained prevention managers who match the local conditions. The organizing institution of such a PM training course needs to know who will be invited to take the course, where they are going to offer their newly acquired skills (or where are they going to implement the idea of primary prevention), what their basic qualifications are, and what their tasks will be in the process of implementing and performing diabetes prevention interventions. With this knowledge, and a realistic estimation of the extent of social and political appreciation and support for diabetes prevention, a structured training program can be planned and defined – or adapted to local needs if an existing model curriculum (like the IMAGE curriculum) is used as a basic version.

Traditionally, a curriculum in the context of teaching and training defines:
- Learning objectives;
- Teaching methods; and
- Didactical materials.

Learning objectives define what the target group of the learning process is supposed to know or to achieve (during or) at the end of the respective training module; so learning objectives describe observable student behavior or performance; a learning objective does not describe the teaching method of the trainer nor the intended level of trainee attention or conduct/obedience in the classroom.

Learning objectives have at least three components:
1. The subject or the target group of the teaching process, which in this case is the PM^{T2Dm}. So, the first part of a learning objective in a curriculum for the training of prevention managers reads: "At the end of this training module the PM^{T2Dm} trainee should be able to . . .".
2. The object of instruction: this is the topic or the content the particular (sub) unit of the training process deals with (e.g., tasks of the prevention manager); and
3. The behavior defining how the trainee is supposed to act (e.g., to describe, to explain, to calculate, to distinguish, to point out, to analyse, to present) in respect of the object or content.

Examples of this are; "At the end of this training module the PM^{T2Dm} trainee should be able to. . .":
- name the tasks of the prevention manager;
- know the data on increasing prevalence of type 2 diabetes in the world and in the trainee's own country;
- explain the evidence for interventions to prevent type 2 diabetes.

Additional optional components of a learning objective are the definition of a condition (such as a specific situation, prerequisite, or aid), a defined detailed content or performance criteria.

The majority of the learning objectives for prevention managers belong to the cognitive domain aiming at the knowledge to be acquired.

Bloom [12,13] created a taxonomy of learning objective levels because the skills in the cognitive domain range from gaining knowledge to critical thinking and making judgments. There are six levels in Bloom's taxonomy, moving through the lowest order processes to the highest:

Knowledge → Comprehension → Application
→ Analysis → Synthesis → Evaluation

The behavioral verbs of the learning objectives at a certain level have to meet the intended complexity of the cognitive learning process:
- Basic level of knowledge: to state, to list, to memorize;
- Comprehension: to explain, to give examples, to illustrate;
- Application: to prepare, to sketch;
- Analysis: to compare, to distinguish;
- Synthesis: to produce, to develop, to design;
- Evaluation: to judge, to recommend.

This differentiation of taxonomy levels should be considered in the development of learning objectives.

The other two domains of learning objectives are "psychomotor" (doing; e.g., participants of the patient education program (persons with hypertension) should be able to perform self-monitoring of their blood pressure correctly) and "affective" (feeling and responsibility; e.g., participants of the patient education program (persons with type 1 diabetes) should be able to express and discuss their feelings and concerns about nighttime hypoglycemia).

In English, the terms "goal" and "objective" are often used interchangeably. In the curriculum context the term "learning goal" is currently preferred for the description of a superior, general outcome of a training module; the "learning objective" is used for the description of more specific subordinate objectives. In other languages there is just one term for goal and objective, like the word *Ziel* in German. Semantic differences become clearer with adjectives such as major learning objectives (=learning goals) and specific learning objectives.

A method to structure the components of the curriculum is to describe the major learning goals in the head sector of the curriculum of the module and define the specific learning objectives, the corresponding teaching methods, and the didactical material in a table of three columns.

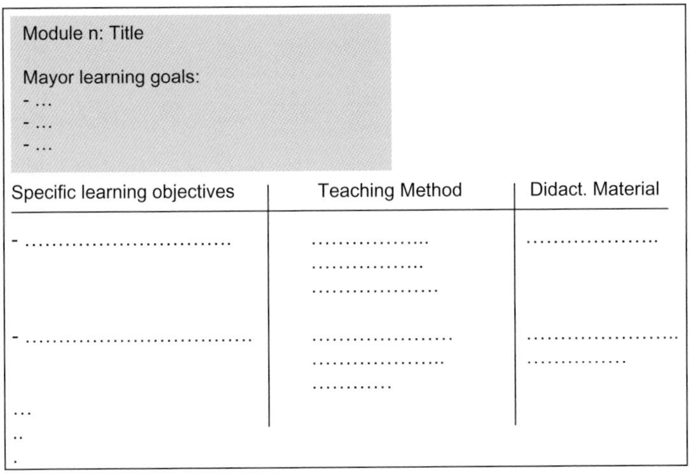

Figure 10.2 Proposal for a schematic pattern to define learning goals/objectives, teaching method, and didactical materials as a core component of structured education.

Usually, the "specific learning objectives" are listed in the left-hand column; they are accompanied by the description of proposed "teaching methods" (middle column), and "materials/media" (right-hand column) (Figure 10.2).

In the column "teaching method," the educational procedures and actions of the lecturer of the didactical unit in order to achieve the respective specific learning objective are described. This description contains action verbs (e.g., "explain," "ask," "collect the responses," "summarize," "distribute") and the content with details what has to be explained, asked, or distributed.

The proposed corresponding didactical material and media (e.g., slides, charts, handouts, worksheets) are defined and listed in the right-hand column. The extended versions of these media should be attached to each part of the curriculum as an appendix in the form of PowerPoint or pdf documents.

An example of a page from the curriculum for prevention managers developed in the context of the IMAGE project is shown in Figure 10.3.

Control of learning objectives

Traditional forms of controlling learning objectives are oral or written exams at the end of the learning process. These focus on the control of

Specific Learning Objectives At the end of the training unit, the prevention manager should...	Teaching Methods	Didactical Material / Media

PA9.1: ... state different techniques to assess physical <u>activity</u>.	**Explain** (by using Chart PA37 and showing devices):
	
	Techniques to assess physical activity (levels):
	  - Self report questionnaires (**e.g.** International Physical Activity Questionnaire - IPAQ)
	  - Physical activity diaries
	  - Activity monitors (e.g. pedometers, accelerometers)
	  - Motion sensors
	  - heart rate monitors
		Chart PA37
		[Techniques to assess physical activities]
		
		Handout: (inter)national PA assessment questionnaires – e.g. IPAQ or PA diaries
		
		Devices for demonstrations, such as pedometer, accelerometer, heart rate monitors

PA9.2: ... give examples for different methods to assess and evaluate physical <u>fitness</u>.	**Lecture on** objective indicators for physical fitness such as
	  - **fitness tests** to assess endurance, strength and flexibility abilities.
	  - Maximum heart rate by treadmill test
	  - VO_{2max} if a lab is available
	
	Explain (by using Chart PA38):
	Suggestions for a **unified fitness** test:
	  a) Endurance: 6-Minutes Walking Test (UKK 2-km-Walking-Test alternatively)
	  b) Strength: Sit-up, Push-up, Standing long jump test
	  c) Coordination: Balance Test (Flamingo Balance Test)
	  d) Flexibility: Sit and Reach
	
	Explain:
	The use of valid test instruments is necessary to guarantee scientific demands and standards. In practice they should be used as a motivational tool (comparing pre and post course result on individual basis). Hint: all the test items will be demonstrated in detail in the following practical learning unit.
		Chart PA38
		[Techniques to assess physical fitness]

Figure 10.3 A 1-page example from the IMAGE curriculum for prevention managers from Module 4: Specific aspects of physical activity in diabetes prevention.

cognitive aspects of the training. With a given major goal to implement diabetes prevention in a local health care setting, this management component can be assessed by an individual longitudinal project report (see Module 7 in the IMAGE PM training) capable of serving as the final thesis of the training program. Such a longitudinal project report should reveal the respective implementation activities describing the following:

- Steps of implementation of the prevention program;
- Intervention team and facilities;
- Methods and contents of the prevention program;
- Concepts of recruitment and networking; and
- Evaluation instruments as well as collected preliminary evaluation data, if available.

This type of control instrument focuses on organization and management activities of the trainee and may be useful during the difficult phase of implementing diabetes prevention.

Each institution responsible for carrying out prevention manager training will define the means of learning process control, probably combining various methods. With the aim of establishing a nationally accepted certificate for the prevention manager, national regulations and conditions have to be respected. Those regulations for accreditation and certifying training and study programs can influence examination conditions as well as contact hours and credits for the whole learning process, the qualification for the lecturers, and the entrance qualifications for the trainees.

The PM training course

The national organizer of prevention manager training will document the basic situation and conditions for the establishment of type 2 diabetes prevention interventions (see earlier) and name experts in the respective scientific fields of prevention to work upon a national curriculum for PM training. Such a curriculum can be developed individually, which is an enormously time-consuming process, or existing curricula can be used as references and a basis to build upon. Within the IMAGE project, a proposed version of a PM training curriculum was developed and disseminated in English [4,5]; the national experts took the developed English version of the corresponding materials and documents, carried out the necessary national adaptations, and arranged for the translation of the material into their own languages.

A formal trainee certification process has to be defined and incorporated into the whole concept and then the time structure and place of the training course, the number of participants and further organizational aspects of the course (e.g., costs, catering) have to be arranged.

An important question to answer is whether and which decision makers should be invited to the PM training course – as a regular participant, as a guest or speaker? Experiences from some countries show that the inclusion of these people into the training program may support its implementation and increase awareness for the need for diabetes prevention activities.

In diabetes treatment the widespread appreciation of education programs took more than half a century – the establishment of qualified and certified prevention manager training can substantially support the implementation of structured prevention programs for persons at risk in a somewhat shorter timeframe.

References

1. Joslin EP. The routine treatment of diabetes with insulin. JAMA 1923;80:1581–3.

2. Joslin EP. The Treatment of Diabetes Mellitus, 3rd edn. Philadelphia/New York: Lea & Febiger; 1923: p. 60.

3. Ahmad LA, Crandall JP. Type 2 diabetes prevention: a review. Clin Diabetes 2010;28:53–9.

4. Kronsbein P, Fischer MR, Tolks D, Greaves C, Puhl S, Stych KE, et al.; on behalf of the IMAGE Study Group. IMAGE: Development of a European curriculum for the training of prevention managers. Br J Diabetes Vasc Dis 2011;11:163–7.

5. Kronsbein P, for the IMAGE Study Group. IMAGE project: curriculum for the training of prevention managers – Type 2 diabetes. Br J Diabetes Vasc Dis 2011; 11(Suppl 2).

6. Spitzenverband GKV. Leitfaden Prävention. Handlungsfelder und Kriterien des GKV-Spitzenverbandes zur Umsetzung von §§ 20 und 20a SGB V vom 21. Juni 2000 in der Fassung vom 27. August 2010. 2. korrigierte Fassung vom 10. November 2010. gkv-press.

7. Oberlinner C, Neumann SM, Ott MG, Zober A. Screening for pre-diabetes and diabetes in the workplace. Occup Med (Lond) 2008;58:41–5.

8. World Health Organization (WHO). Occupational health. Workplace health promotion. 2012. Available from: www.who.int/occupational_health/topics/workplace/en/ (accessed 9 March 2013).

9. van Dongen JM, Proper KI, van Wier MF, van der Beek AJ, Bongers PM, van Mechelen W, et al. Systematic review on the financial return of workside health promotion programmes aimed at improving nutrition and/or increasing physical activity. Obes Rev 2011;12:1031–49.

10. Ackermann RT, Finch EA, Brizendine E, Zhou H, Marrero DG. Translating the diabetes prevention program into the community: The DEPLOY Pilot Study. Am J Prev Med 2008;35:357–63.

11. Finch EA, Kelly MS, Marrero DG, Ackermann RT. Training YMCA wellness instructors to deliver an adapted version of the Diabetes Prevention Program lifestyle intervention. Diabetes Educ 2009;35:224–32.

12. Bloom BS. Taxonomy of educational objectives: the classification of educational goals. Handbook I: Cognitive domain. New York: David McKay Co.; 1969.

13. Anderson LW, Krathwohl DR, editors. Taxonomy of Learning, Teaching, and Assessing: A Revision of Bloom's Taxonomy of Educational Objectives. New York/San Fransisco/Boston: Longman; 2001.

CHAPTER 11

Prevention of type 2 diabetes: the role of physical activity

Thomas Yates[1,2], Melanie Davies[1,2] and Kamlesh Khunti[1]

[1] Diabetes Research Unit, College of Medicine, Biological Sciences and Psychology, University of Leicester, Leicester, UK
[2] National Institute for Health Research Leicester – Loughborough Diet, Lifestyle and Physical Activity Biomedical Research Unit, University Hospitals of Leicester and University of Leicester, Leicester, UK

Physical activity and health – an evolutionary perspective

Physical activity, referring to bodily movement requiring energy expenditure produced by skeletal muscles, is innately involved in the regulation of metabolic health in humans. The human phenotype is highly sensitive to alterations in the amount of physical activity conducted, particularly outside the bounds of those considered physiologically normal; for example, severe metabolic dysfunction develops when physical movement is limited to bed rest. Therefore, the high levels of physical inactivity associated with modern daily life are one of the fundamental drivers of the modern epidemic of type 2 diabetes. The underlying reason for this can only be fully understood by considering Dobzhansky's famous maxim that "nothing in biology makes sense except in the light of evolution" [1].

Historically, the survival of the species depended on the ability to adapt to environmental change over time. Modern humans evolved during the Palaeolithic period, which began approximately 2.6 million years ago and ended 10000 years ago [2]. It has been suggested that the emerging human lineage was forced to adapt to withstand ever-increasing amounts of daily physical activity due to environmental pressures and the emergence of a bipedal gait, which favored endurance over power and speed [2]. Regardless of the underlying evolution drivers, it is clear that humans evolved into highly adapted hunter-gatherers whose primary weapon was the ability to withstand epic feats of endurance rarely witnessed in the

Prevention of Diabetes, First Edition. Edited by Peter Schwarz and Prasuna Reddy.
© 2013 John Wiley & Sons, Ltd. Published 2013 by John Wiley & Sons, Ltd.

animal kingdom. This is typified by persistence hunting, thought to have been practiced by our hunter-gatherer ancestors and documented over the last century in some of the few remaining nomadic tribes [3]. Persistence hunting refers to a hunting strategy that entails relentlessly tracking faster animals, such as antelope or deer, for mile after mile, allowing the animal little opportunity to rest, until it eventually overheats and collapses with exhaustion. In addition to the high energy cost of hunting, persistence or otherwise, there were a plethora of other essential daily activities that would have incurred a substantial energy cost, from scouring the surrounding environment for additional sources of edible fuel, to carrying infants (the average child was estimated to be carried 1500 km during its first 2 years of life [2]), to securing shelter, to name but a few. On a metabolic level, this continual demand for high levels of physical activity would have favored alleles that were associated with optimal function in such environments [4,5].

While the emergence of agriculture around 10000 years ago had a dramatic effect on the structure of human society and profoundly changed the way food was produced, high levels of physical activity would still have been inextricably linked to food procurement for the majority of the population [6,7]. Not until the advent of the Industrial Revolution did our lifestyle slowly start to become discordant with our evolved physiology, a process that occurred with particular rapidity in the second half of the twentieth century.

We now live in an environment that is totally divorced from that in which we evolved; indeed, we have reached a point where all the necessities of modern life such as working, shopping, banking, socialization, and entertainment can be fulfilled while sitting in front of a screen. Therefore, unsurprisingly, modern society is characterized by high levels of physical inactivity. A modern office worker is estimated to meet only one-third of the energy expenditure needed to survive in hunter-gatherer conditions and objective assessments classify 95% of the population in industrialized societies as inactive through failing to meet the minimum recommendations for health [3,8,9].

The direct result of breaking the link between hard physical labor and food procurement has been an unprecedented epidemic of metabolic dysfunction characterized by high levels of obesity and chronic disease. Physical inactivity is associated with over 20 diseases and conditions and is now estimated by the World Health Organization to be the fourth leading cause of premature mortality globally, ahead of both obesity and dietary factors [10,11]. Others have shown that low levels cardiorespiratory fitness, an objective indicator of physical inactivity, is the leading cause of mortality, ahead of both obesity and smoking [12]. Physical inactivity therefore exerts a staggering economic burden on health care systems and economic productivity; for example, the direct and indirect cost of physical inactivity on health care expenditure and the economy in England, United Kingdom, has been estimated at over £8 billion annually [13].

Evidence for the role of physical activity in the prevention of type 2 diabetes

The decreasing levels of physical activity witnessed in modern societies coincided with a dramatic increase in the incidence of type 2 diabetes; for example, a sixfold increase in the prevalence of the disease is estimated to have occurred in the latter half of the twentieth century [10]. Importantly, it is now well established that the link between decreased physical activity and increased prevalence of type 2 diabetes is more than just historical coincidence but is directly related, with the former being one of the primary causal factors of the latter. Indeed, somewhat rarely for lifestyle factors, evidence for a causal link between physical activity and the prevention of type 2 diabetes is supported by the full spectrum of evidence needed to infer causality, from observational research to experimental mechanistic investigation and randomized controlled trials.

Prospective observational research has consistently demonstrated that undertaking levels of physical activity that are consistent with the current physical recommendations for health are associated with a 30–50% reduction in the relative risk of developing type 2 diabetes when compared with those who are inactive [14].

Mechanistic studies have identified multiple pathways linking physical activity to improved glucose transport [15–17]. For example, acute and long-term changes in insulin action and fuel utilization occur through mitochondrial biogenesis, increased fatty acid oxidation, and increased expression and translocation of key signaling proteins involved in the insulin-mediated glucose uptake pathway, particularly GLUT-4 [15]. Interestingly, muscular contractions are also known to induce glucose update through insulin independent pathways, which are likely to involve the upregulation of AMP-activated kinase [16].

Finally, randomized controlled trials and meta-analyses have demonstrated that physical activity interventions result in improved glucose regulation and a reduced risk of diabetes in those with a high risk of the disease [18,19]. For example, an exercise intervention in those with impaired glucose tolerance was shown to reduce 2-hour post-challenge glucose values by 1.3 mmol/L over 12 months and reduce the risk of type 2 diabetes by 60% over 24 months [19,20]. This is consistent with other studies and the results of a meta-analysis demonstrate that physical activity interventions result in around 50% reduction in the relative risk of type 2 diabetes and are as effective as other multi-factorial interventions that also promoted a healthy diet and weight loss [18].

How much is enough?

General physical activity recommendations for adults have typically specified engaging in at least 150 minutes per week of moderate to vigorous intensity physical activity. This weekly target has traditionally been packaged as needing to achieve least 30 minutes on at least 5 days a week in bouts of at least 10 minutes in length. However, recent updated recommendations have started to emphasize and prioritize the weekly (150 minutes) rather than daily (30 minutes) target, allowing more flexibility throughout the week in how the recommendations are accumulated [21,22], although the minimum bout length of 10 minutes still applies. In order to count towards weekly targets, physical activity needs to be undertaken to at least a level of moderate intensity. This is commonly quantified in terms of metabolic equivalents (METs). METs denote intensity as a multiple of the resting metabolic rate. For example, sitting quietly watching television is assigned a MET value of 1, while running is assigned a MET value of 10 or higher, depending on the pace [23]; this can be conceptualized as running requires at least 10 times more energy than sitting per unit of time. A MET value of at least 3 is taken to count as moderate intensity, while a value of greater than 6 is taken to count as vigorous intensity [23]. Table 11.1 highlights common activities and their relative MET values.

In addition to aerobic exercise, national and international physical activity recommendations also recognize the added value to metabolic and functional health of optimizing fat-free body mass by incorporating regular resistance exercise into weekly physical activity routines [21,22]. This does not necessarily require access to gym environments, but can involve simple home-based exercise such as push-ups, sit-ups, and squats with handheld weights, such as food cans or water containers, to increase resistance as necessary.

Table 11.1 Common activities and their associated MET levels.

Intensity level	Activity	MET level
Sedentary	Reclining – reading a book/newspaper	1.0
	Sitting – quietly watching TV	1.0
	Sitting – reading a book/newspaper	1.3
	Sitting – talking on phone	1.5
	Sitting – eating	1.5
	Sitting – light office work	1.5
Light intensity	Standing – talking, reading a book, etc.	1.8
activities	Walking – slow, 2 mph	2.0
	Cooking	2.0
Moderate	Walking – brisk, 3 mph	3.3
intensity activities	Walking – moderate effort carrying infant or 4.5 kg load	3.5
	Vacuuming/mopping floor – continuous effort	3.5
	Gardening – general	4.0
	Bicycling – <10 mph	4.0
	Golf – general, walking and carry clubs	4.5
	Badminton	4.5
	Walking – fast, 4 mph	5.0
	Bicycling – 10–11.9 mph	6.0
	Swimming – general	6.0
Vigorous	Walking – very fast, 4.5 mph	6.3
intensity activities	Jogging	7.0
	Bicycling – 12–13.9 mph	8.0
	Running – 6 mph	10.0
	Swimming – fast, vigorous effort	10.0
	Running – 8 mph	13.5

Source: derived from Ainsworth et al. [23].

Recommendations specifically aimed at the prevention of type 2 diabetes have not been formally developed or specified. However, it is unlikely that such recommendations would differ substantially from those developed for the general population, as successful diabetes prevention programs and exercise intervention in those at high risk of type 2 diabetes have consistently promoted levels that are consistent with 150 minutes of moderate to vigorous intensity physical activity per week [24,25]. Furthermore, given that glucose regulation exists on a continuous rather than categorical spectrum, inferences can also be drawn from recommendations for those with type 2 diabetes. For example, the American Diabetes

Association recommends that individuals with type 2 diabetes should perform aerobic exercise of at least moderate intensity in bouts of at least 10 minutes on at least 3 days per week (with no more than 2 consecutive days between bouts) accumulating a total of at least 150 minutes per week [26]. Furthermore, in terms of glucose control, it has been found that those with relatively worse glucose regulation, whether through impaired glucose regulation or type 2 diabetes, get the greatest benefit from undertaking physical activity interventions, demonstrating that those with worse glucose control have the most to gain from undertaking physical activity [27,28].

It should also be emphasized that the promoted target of 150 minutes per week is a minimum level needed to achieve some health benefits. However, national and international recommendations now specifically state that greater benefits will be gained through achieving higher volumes of physical activity [21,22]. This can either be achieved by increasing the intensity level of the activity undertaken or by increasing the time spent in moderate intensity activity, or both. This is likely to be particularly relevant for the prevention of type 2 diabetes where epidemiologic evidence has consistently demonstrated a dose–response relationship between the amount of physical activity undertaken and the risk of type 2 diabetes [14]. A recent meta-analysis of physical activity interventions in those with type 2 diabetes also reported that both frequency and total duration of physical activity undertaken were significantly associated with greater glycemic improvements; those achieving more than 150 minutes per week gaining the most benefit [27].

In summary, individuals identified at high risk of diabetes, either by the presence of impaired glucose regulation or with known risk factors, should aim to achieve at least 150 minutes of moderate to vigorous intensity physical activity per week and that higher levels above this minimum target will convey greater benefit.

Physical activity and body weight

Given that physical activity is one of the key determinants of energy expenditure, physical activity is indelibly associated with weight loss in the wider public and health care professional conscience. Therefore, interventions aimed at physical activity behavior change are often judged by their success or failure at initiating weight loss. This is particularly true in type 2 diabetes given the close link to obesity.

However, linking the effectiveness of physical activity interventions to weight loss is misleading and likely to be counterproductive. There is overwhelming evidence, supported by numerous adiposity independent mechanisms [15,16], that increased physical activity promotes metabolic health and improves glycemic control independent of weight loss [17]. For example, an intervention study in overweight and obese individuals at high risk of type 2 diabetes demonstrated substantial improvements in glucose regulation following an exercise intervention despite no significant change to body weight or waist circumference [19,20]. Similarly, the Indian Diabetes Prevention Program reported significant reductions in the relative risk of type 2 diabetes following a lifestyle intervention, largely focused on the promotion of physical activity, despite no change to body weight of the participants [29]. This finding is consistent with data from the Finnish Diabetes Prevention Study which reported that those who walked for 150 minutes per week had over 50% reduced relative risk of type 2 diabetes compared with those who walked for less than 1 hour per week, after adjustment for adiposity and dietary intake [30]. Meta-analyses have also shown that weight loss did not explain observed improvements in glycemic control following an exercise intervention in those with type 2 diabetes [27,31].

Increased physical activity is also known to alter the distribution of body fat without affecting overall body weight. For example, exercise training has been shown to reduce visceral and hepatic adipose tissue without impacting on overall weight [32]. High levels of visceral and hepatic adipose tissue have a profoundly deleterious impact on metabolic regulation regardless of overall body fat. Therefore, upon initiation of increased physical activity, individuals may undergo positive alterations to their fat distribution and metabolic health, but experience no discernable change to their body weight. This is typified by sumo wrestlers who, while training, have normal levels of visceral adiposity and are metabolically healthy despite high levels of total body fat; it is only upon retirement and the cessation of training that ill health manifests itself [33].

Crucially, when considering the interplay between these factors, it is well established that achieving levels of physical activity that are consistent with the minimum recommendations for health is unlikely to result in meaningful weight loss. Recent physical activity recommendation advice that around 60 minutes per day of moderate intensity physical activity is needed to initiate and maintain weight loss [21,22]. This has important implications because it means that those attempting physical activity behavior change as a method of losing weight are likely to become demotivated and revert to a sedentary lifestyle if their desired end-product is not achieved, despite gaining other, more clinically relevant, health benefits such as improved glucose regulation.

Therefore it is clear that the promotion of physical activity significantly improves metabolic health, even in the absence of weight loss, and that the historic preoccupation of judging physical activity behavior change with weight loss needs to challenged, both among health care professionals and the general public, in order for physical activity to be utilized to its full potential. This message will find resonance with many sections of society who have tried and failed to lose weight on numerous occasions; shifting the emphasis away from body image to a positive message of embracing a healthy lifestyle for its own sake is often met with enthusiasm and relief.

Promotion of physical activity in diabetes prevention: what works

Physical activity is a complex behavior that is determined by host of different multi-level factors from individual to societal. In modern industrialized environments, most of these factors now act to discourage healthful levels of physical activity. Therefore, the first task is to recognize that changing physical activity levels is likely to require substantial effort on the part of participants and a rigorous evidence-based framework on behalf of health care professionals – simply providing brief advice and informing individuals that they should be more active, as is the case in many health care consultations, is ineffectual. As with other lifestyle behaviors, physical activity promotion in high-risk populations needs to involve robust motivational and volitional elements.

Motivational elements include increasing knowledge of diabetes and diabetes risk and how this can be ameliorated by physical activity, self-efficacy for behavior change, and discussion of potential barriers and how they can be overcome [34]. In general, motivational factors can be considered as those that increase one's intention to change behavior. Volitional elements are used to convert intention into action and include self-regulatory strategies such as setting personalized goals, forming action plans detailing where, when, and how the planned activity will take place, and self-monitoring performance [34–36]. Traditional frameworks and theories for promoting behavior change, such as the theory of planned behavior, have typically under-utilized volitional aspects and hence have had limited success [37,38]. This is particularly true of physical activity where, given the complexity of issues involved, establishing successful strategies for self-regulating behavior is essential. This concept can be usefully illustrated and explored with pedometer (step counter) use.

Pedometers

Walking is now commonly acknowledged to be the preferred choice of physical activity in free-living environments for both the general population and those at high risk of type 2 diabetes and is therefore likely to form the focus of diabetes prevention initiatives [39]. Pedometers form a powerful self-regulatory tool in the promotion of walking activity as they raise awareness of current activity levels, provide objective feedback to the wearer, and facilitate clear and simple goal setting. Interventions based on pedometer use have been shown to be highly successful at promoting increased physical activity in multiple populations [40]. However, in order to be effective, realistic and personalized step-per-day goals are needed that take account of current activity levels; generic goals that are too ambitious can be demotivating and lead to failure. This is particularly relevant to those with a high risk of chronic disease who are likely to start from a lower base than the general population; indeed, the commonly promoted 10 000 steps per day target could easily represent a tripling of usual activity levels in a large proportion of this population.

In the first instance, sedentary individuals should be helped to determine their baseline levels of activity and then aim for an average increase in ambulatory activity of around 2000 steps per day which should be undertaken in a purposeful manner (i.e., at moderate intensity). An increase of this magnitude represents around 20 minutes per day of increased moderate walking activity and is therefore roughly equivalent to the current recommendations of 150 minutes of moderate intensity activity per week [41]. This distal goal should be broken down into several proximal steps, such as an increase of 500 steps every fortnight. This approach has proven highly successful in promoting long-term increases to physical activity and improved glucose regulation in those with a high risk of type 2 diabetes [19,20].

Categories of ambulatory activity, highlighted and summarized in Table 11.2, have also been proposed to aid public health initiatives and interventions incorporating pedometers. Here the first propriety should be to help individuals move up to a high activity category.

Table 11.2 Physical activity categories based on steps per day.

Category	Steps per day
Sedentary	<5000
Low: typical of daily activity excluding volitional activity	5000–7499
Moderate: likely to incorporate the equivalent of around 30 minutes per day of moderate intensity physical activity	7500–9999
High: likely to incorporate the equivalent of around 45 minutes per day of moderate intensity physical activity	10000–12499
Very high: likely to incorporate the equivalent of over 45 minutes per day of moderate intensity physical activity	>12500

Source: adapted from Tudor-Locke and Bassett [41].

In summary, incorporating effective self-regulatory strategies, such as pedometer use, are of primary importance in the promoting of physical activity and should not be overshadowed by motivational elements.

Physical activity and the detection of risk

Although physical inactivity is recognized as one of the most important modifiable risk factors in the prevention of type 2 diabetes, it has limited utility in helping to identify and rank risk through inclusion in risk scores or other risk stratification methods; this is for several important reasons. First, physical inactivity is a near-universal condition. It has consistently been shown that 50–80% of the population in both developed and developing countries fail to meet the minimum recommendations for health [42–44]; when physical activity levels are measured objectively, this figure rises to 95% [8,9]. Second, methods that rely on individuals self-reporting their activity levels are highly inaccurate and unreliable. For example, a commonly used and internationally validated self-reported measure of physical activity describes as little as 10% of the variation in objectively measure levels [45]; this is in contrast to simple measures of adiposity, such as body mass index (BMI), which are reasonably accurate on a population level and hence provide a powerful discriminator of diabetes risk.

For these reasons, commonly used definitions or measures of physical inactivity do not provide a clear mechanism for stratifying diabetes risk and do not therefore add to the predictive power of diabetes risk scores.

However, although of limited academic importance in the classification of diabetes risk, it is still important that physical activity assessment is included in tools that are routinely used to help individuals self-assess their level of diabetes risk. This is because most factors, apart from measures of adiposity, that significantly contribute to commonly used diabetes risk scores are non-modifiable through lifestyle change, such as age, family history of diabetes, sex, and medication status [46]. Therefore, on undertaking a self-assessment of diabetes risk, it will not be apparent that the individual's future risk of diabetes can be substantially modified by lifestyle factors. Moreover, even if an individual was motivated to change their lifestyle as a result of discovering they were at a high risk of type 2 diabetes, the fact that such changes are not mirrored by a lowering of their assessed risk is likely to be demotivating and counterproductive. For these reasons, FINDRISC, one of the most commonly used and widely validated self-assessment diabetes risk scores, includes physical activity in the quantification of diabetes risk [46].

Physical activity throughout life

Although chronic disease was once thought to only affect older adults, it is now recognized that the general increase in harmful lifestyle behaviors, including low levels of physical activity, has been mirrored in younger populations over the last couple of decades and is driving a substantial shift in the demographic profile of some chronic diseases. Type 2 diabetes is the starkest demonstration of this phenomenon; prevalence rates in younger adults and children (<40 years) have increased by up to 10-fold over recent decades, with dramatic effects on the risk of cardiovascular morbidity and mortality in this population [47]. As with adults, there is good evidence that levels of physical activity are strongly and inversely associated with metabolic health in children and adolescents [48–50], suggesting that physical inactivity is a central factor driving the changing demographic of disease in this population. Therefore it is vitally important that physical activity levels are promoted and sustained throughout the life course. Physical activity levels in adolescence are particularly important as they determine the peak levels of cardiorespiratory fitness and skeletal muscle power achieved in one's lifetime [51]. Higher peak lifetime values in these factors provide an elevated point from which natural and unavoidable functional declines due to aging occur [51]. This has clinical consequences as higher peak levels and higher absolute values throughout the life-course delay the onset of physical frailty and reduce the risk of morbidity and premature mortality [51–53]. The discrepancies between a lifetime of physical activity and inactivity are so extreme that individuals who are highly active throughout their life will have a higher level of cardiorespiratory fitness when they are 75 years old than an obese inactive individual may ever achieve [54]. However, it should be emphasized that the consequences of a history of inactivity can be ameliorated to a certain extent with increased activity at any point throughout the life course [51]. However, unless effectively targeted, the increasing levels of inactivity in younger generations are storing up a tidal wave of metabolic dysfunction, illness, and under-productivity in later years that will have a startling effect on the economic potential of future generations and greatly increase the accompanying health care burden.

Sedentary behavior: more than just physical inactivity

Over the last decade there has been increasing attention to the role that sedentary behavior has on metabolic health, independent of other factors including moderate to vigorous intensity physical activity. Indeed, sedentary behavior is now widely considered a separate paradigm with independent determinants and effects on metabolic health [55–57]. Sedentary behavior is broadly defined as tasks requiring a metabolic equivalent (MET) of 1.5 or less (Table 11.1) [58]. However, this technical definition can be operationally defined as non-exercise activities conducted while sitting. When sitting or lying, the majority of the body's largest muscle groups are relaxed; in contrast, when standing, even if relatively still, a large proportion of the body's musculature is under tension and energy expenditure is commonly above the 1.5 MET sedentary threshold. Under this operational definition, any standing activity can be considered non-sedentary. In this context, sedentary behavior defines a different behavior context than physical inactivity; the latter is commonly conceptualized as failing to meet the physical activity guidelines for health or not engaging in any moderate to vigorous levels of physical activity. Thus, it is possible to be undertaking non-sedentary activity, such as engaging in low-intensity ambulatory activity, while being technically inactive. This distinction may seem subtle, but it has important consequences that could revolutionize the content of diabetes prevention programs in the future.

There is now mounting epidemiological and experimental evidence that the amount of time spent in sitting-related sedentary behaviors and the number of times sedentary behavior is broken throughout the day are associated with the risk of insulin resistance and type 2 diabetes independent of physical activity [59–61]; the higher the total time spent sedentary, the higher the risk and conversely the greater the number of breaks to sedentary behavior, such as transitioning from sitting to standing, the lower the risk. Importantly, emerging observational research also suggests that incorporating the recommended amount of physical activity into an otherwise sedentary lifestyle does not fully ameliorate the risks associated with high levels of sitting-related sedentary behavior [62,63]. These observations are consistent with animal models that have demonstrated that distinctive mechanisms around the action of lipoprotein-lipase that respond to increased sedentary behavior on an order of magnitude great than they do increased physical activity [55]. These findings suggest that amount of time spent sitting throughout the day could be a key independent lifestyle-related driver of the modern epidemic of type 2 diabetes, regardless of the amount of moderate to vigorous intensity conducted and that, conversely, prevention programs that do not take these findings into account may fail to maximize their potential effectiveness. For instance, individuals could be encouraged to substitute a proportion of their sitting time during common leisure and work-related activities for standing. Simple strategies could include advocating standing during advert breaks when watching TV, constructing and utilizing standing stations for computerized work, and holding meetings while standing [57]. However, while the epidemiologic evidence base to date is strong enough to necessitate the attention of interventionists and policy markers, there is currently a lack of interventional level evidence in humans which negates the ability to make any firm recommendations or conclusions. Therefore, it is vitally important that programs that incorporate messages around reductions in sedentary time do not deflect focus from those aimed at the promotion of increased moderate to vigorous intensity physical activity, but work together synergistically.

Conclusions

This chapter presents evidence demonstrating that low levels of physical activity are one of the most important, if not the most important, lifestyle factors driving the current epidemic of type 2 diabetes witnessed in all corners of the globe. We evolved to have a physiology that is uniquely adapted to withstand, and achieve optimal metabolic health through, high levels of physical activity related energy expenditure. It is clear that the multiple modern barriers to, and inducements against, living out this heritage have left a trail of metabolic dysfunction in its wake at both the individual and societal level. Conversely, there is clear and consistent evidence, from all levels needed to confirm direction of causality, that increased physical activity can substantially lower insulin resistance and the risk of type 2 diabetes. Therefore, the promotion of increased physical activity should be one of the primary focuses of any diabetes prevention initiative. It is also vital that efforts to promote physical activity are not judged, either by health care professionals or patients, through the effect on body weight or commonly used indices of adiposity such as BMI, but by a more holistic definition of health and well-being. In short, physical activity, more than any other single lifestyle behavior, needs to take center stage if we are to achieve a step change in the battle against type 2 diabetes.

References

1. Dobzhansky T. Nothing in biology makes sense except in the light of evolution. Am Biol Teacher 1973;35:125–9.
2. Cordain L, Gotshall RW, Eaton SB, Eaton SB 3rd. Physical activity, energy expenditure and fitness: an evolutionary perspective. Int J Sports Med 1998;19:328–35.
3. Liebenberg L. Persistence hunting by modern hunter-gatherers. Curr Anthropol 2006;47:1017–25.
4. Chakravarthy M, Booth F. Eating, exercise, and "thrifty" genotypes: connecting the dots toward an evolutionary understanding of modern chronic diseases. J Appl Phsiol 2004;96:3–10.
5. Booth F, Chakravarthy M, Spangenburg E. Exercise and gene expression: physiological regulation of the human genome through physical activity. J Physiol 2002;543:399–411.
6. Egger GJ, Vogels N, Westerterp KR. Estimating historical changes in physical activity levels. Med J Aust 2001;175:635–6.
7. James WP. A public health approach to the problem of obesity. Int J Obes Relat Metab Disord 1995;19(Suppl 3):S37–45.
8. NHS Information Centre. Health survey for England, 2008: physical activity and fitness. 2009. Available from: www.ic.nhs.uk/statistics-and-data-collections/health-and-lifestyles-related-surveys/health-survey-for-england/health-survey-for-england–2008-physical-activity-and-fitness (accessed 6 March 2013).
9. Troiano RP, Berrigan D, Dodd KW, Mâsse LC, Tilert T, McDowell M. Physical activity in the United States measured by accelerometer. Med Sci Sports Exerc 2008;40:181–8.

10. Booth FW, Gordon SE, Carlson CJ, Hamilton MT. Waging war on modern chronic diseases: primary prevention through exercise biology. J Appl Phsiol 2000;88: 774–87.

11. World Health Organization: Global Health Risks: Mortality and Burden of Disease Attributable to Selected Major Risk Factors. Geneva, Switzerland: World Health Organization, 2009.

12. Blair SN. Physical inactivity: the biggest public health problem of the 21st century. Br J Sports Med 2009;43:1–2.

13. Department of Health. At least five a week: evidence on the impact of physical activity and its relationship to health. 2004; Available at: http://www.dh.gov.uk/en/ Publicationsandstatistics/Publications/PublicationsPolicyAndGuidance/ DH_4080994 (accessed 6 March 2013).

14. Bassuk SS, Manson JE: Epidemiological evidence for the role of physical activity in reducing risk of type 2 diabetes and cardiovascular disease. J Appl Physiol 2005;99: 1193–204.

15. Hawley JA. Exercise as a therapeutic intervention for the prevention and treatment of insulin resistance. Diabetes Metab Res Rev 2004;20:383–93.

16. Hawley JA, Lessard SJ. Exercise training-induced improvements in insulin action. Acta Physiol 2008;192:127–35.

17. Telford RD. Low physical activity and obesity: causes of chronic disease or simply predictors? Med Sci Sports Exerc 2007;39:1233–40.

18. Gillies, CL, Abrams KR, Lambert PC, Cooper NJ, Sutton AJ, Hsu RT, et al. Pharmacological and lifestyle interventions to prevent or delay type 2 diabetes in people with impaired glucose tolerance: systematic review and meta-analysis. BMJ 2007;334:299–308.

19. Yates T, Davies M, Gorely T, Bull F, Khunti K. Effectiveness of a pragmatic education programme aimed at promoting walking activity in individuals with impaired glucose tolerance: a randomized controlled trial. Diabetes Care 2009;32:1404–10.

20. Yates T, Daves M, Sehmi S, Gorely T, Khunti K. The Prediabetes Risk Education and Physical Activity Recommendation and Encouragement (PREPARE) programme study: are improvements in glucose regulation sustained at two years? Diabet Med 2011;10:1268–71.

21. World Health Organization. Global Recommendations on Physical Activity for Health. Geneva, World Health Organization, 2010.

22. Department of Health. Start active, stay active: a report on physical activity from the four home countries' Chief Medical Officers, 2011. Available at http://www. dh.gov.uk/en/Publicationsandstatistics/Publications/PublicationsPolicyAnd Guidance/DH_128209 (accessed 6 March 2013).

23. Ainsworth B, Haskell W, Whitt M, Irwin ML, Swartz AM, Strath SJ, et al. Compendium of Physical Activities: an update of activity codes and MET intensities. Med Sci Sports Exerc 2000;32:S498–516.

24. Tuomilehto J, Lindström J, Eriksson JG, Valle TT, Hämäläinen H, Ilanne-Parikka P, et al. Prevention of type 2 diabetes mellitus by changes in lifestyle among subjects with impaired glucose tolerance. N Engl J Med 2001;344:1343–50.

25. Knowler WC, Barrett-Connor E, Fowler SE, Hamman RF, Lachin JM, Walker EA, et al. Reduction in the incidence of type 2 diabetes with lifestyle intervention or metformin. N Engl J Med 2002;346:393–403.

26. Colberg SR, Sigal RJ, Fernhall B, Regensteiner JG, Blissmer BJ, Rubin RR, et al. American College of Sports Medicine, American Diabetes Association (2010). Exercise and type 2 diabetes: the American College of Sports Medicine and the American Diabetes Association: joint position statement. Diabetes Care 33(12):e147–67.

27. Umpierre D, Ribeiro PA, Kramer CK, Leitão CB, Zucatti AT, Azevedo MJ, et al. Physical activity advice only or structured exercise training and association with HbA1c levels in type 2 diabetes. JAMA 2011;305:1790–9.

28. Jenkins N, Hagberg J. Aerobic training effects on glucose tolerance in prediabetic and normoglycemic humans. Med Sci Sports Exerc 2011;43:2231–40.

29. Ramachandran A, Snehalatha C, Mary S, Mukesh B, Bhaskar AD, Vijay V; Indian Diabetes Prevention Programme (IDPP). The Indian Diabetes Prevention Programme shows that lifestyle modification and metformin prevent type 2 diabetes in Asian Indian subjects with impaired glucose tolerance (IDPP-1). Diabetologia 2006;49: 289–97.

30. Laaksonen DE, Lindström J, Lakka TA, Eriksson JG, Niskanen L, Wikström K, et al. Physical activity in the prevention of type 2 diabetes: the Finnish diabetes prevention study. Diabetes 2005;54:158–65.

31. Boulé NG, Haddad E, Kenny GP, Wells GA, Sigal RJ. Effects of exercise on glycemic control and body mass in type 2 diabetes mellitus: a meta-analysis of controlled clinical trials. JAMA 2001;286:1218–27.

32. Johnson N, Sachinwalla T, Walton D, Smith K, Armstrong A, Thompson MW, et al. Aerobic exercise training reduces hepatic and visceral lipids in obese individuals without weight loss. Hepatology 2009;50:1105–12.

33. Karelis A, St-Pierre D, Conus F, Rabasa-Lhoret R, Poehlman ET. Metabolic and body composition factors in subgroups of obesity: what we know. J Clin Endocrinol Metab 2004;89:2569–75.

34. Bandura A. Social Foundations of Thought and Action: A Social Cognitive Theory. Englewood Cliffs, NJ: Prentice-Hall; 1986.

35. Sniehotta FF, Scholz U, Schwarzer R. Bridging the intention–behaviour gap: planning, self-efficacy, and action control in the adoption and maintenance of physical exercise. Psychol Health 2005;20:143–60.

36. Gollwitzer PM. Implementation intentions: strong effects of simple plans: how can good intentions become effective behavior change strategies? Am Psychologist 1999;54:493–503.

37. Johnston DW, Johnston M, Pollard B, Kinmonth AL, Mant D. Motivation is not enough: prediction of risk behavior following diagnosis of coronary heart disease from the theory of planned behavior. Health Psychol 2004;23:533–8.

38. Brug J, Oenema A, Ferreira I. Theory, evidence and intervention mapping to improve behavior nutrition and physical activity interventions. Int J Behav Nutr Phys Act 2005;2:2.

39. Yates T, Davies M, Gorely T, Bull F, Khunti K. Rationale, design and baseline data from the PREPARE (Pre-diabetes Risk Education and Physical Activity Recommendation and Encouragement) programme study: a randomized controlled trial. Patient Educ Couns 2008;73:264–71.

40. Bravata DM, Smith-Spangler C, Sundaram V, Gienger AL, Lin N, Lewis R, et al. Using pedometers to increase physical activity and improve health: a systematic review. JAMA 2007;298:2296–304.

41. Tudor-Locke C, Bassett DR Jr. How many steps/day are enough? Preliminary pedometer indices for public health. Sports Med 2004;34:1–8.
42. Sisson SB, Katzmarzyk PT. International prevalence of physical activity in youth and adults. Obes Rev 2008;9:606–14.
43. Carlson SA, Fulton JE, Schoenborn CA, Loustalot F. Physical activity trend and prevalence estimates based on the 2008 Physical Activity Guidelines for Americans, National Health Interview Survey 1998–2008. Am J Prev Med 2010;39:305–13.
44. NHS Information Centre. Health survey for England, 2008: physical activity and fitness. 2009. Available from: www.ic.nhs.uk/statistics-and-data-collections/health-and-lifestyles-related-surveys/health-survey-for-england/health-survey-for-england–2008-physical-activity-and-fitness (avvessed 6 March 2013).
45. Craig CL, Marshall AL, Sjöström M, Bauman AE, Booth ML, Ainsworth BE, et al. International physical activity questionnaire: 12-country reliability and validity. Med Sci Sports Exerc 2003;35:1381–95.
46. Lindström J, Tuomilehto J. The diabetes risk score: a practical tool to predict type 2 diabetes risk. Diabetes Care 2003;26:725–31.
47. Wilmot EG, Davies MJ, Yates T, Benhalima K, Lawrence IG, Khunti K. Type 2 diabetes in younger adults: the emerging UK epidemic. Postgrad Med J 2010;86: 711–8.
48. Owen CG, Nightingale CM, Rudnicka AR, Sattar N, Cook DG, Ekelund U, et al. Physical activity, obesity and cardiometabolic risk factors in 9- to 10-year-old UK children of white European, South Asian and black African-Caribbean origin: the Child Heart And health Study in England (CHASE). Diabetologia 2010;53:1620–30.
49. Metcalf B, Voss L, Hosking J, Jeffery AN, Wilkin TJ. Physical activity at the government recommended level and obesity-related health outcomes: a longitudinal study (Early Bird 37). Arch Dis Child 2008;93:772–7.
50. Janssen I, LeBlanc AG. Systematic review of the health benefits of physical activity and fitness in school-aged children and youth. Int J Behav Nutr Phys Act 2010;7:40.
51. Booth F, Laye M, Roberts M. Lifetime sedentary living accelerates some aspects of secondary aging. J Appl Physiol 2011;111:1497–504.
52. Kokkinos P, Myers J. Exercise and physical activity: clinical outcomes and applications. Circulation 2010;122:1637–48.
53. Kodama S, Saito K, Tanaka S, Maki M, Yachi Y, Asumi M, et al. Cardiorespiratory fitness as a quantitative predictor of all-cause mortality and cardiovascular events in healthy men and women: a meta-analysis. JAMA 2009;301:2024–35.
54. Heath GW, Hagberg JM, Ehsani AA, Holloszy JO. A physiological comparison of young and older endurance athletes. J Appl Physiol 1981;51:634–40.
55. Hamilton MT, Hamilton DG, Zderic TW. Role of low energy expenditure and sitting in obesity, metabolic syndrome, type 2 diabetes, and cardiovascular disease. Diabetes 2007;56:2655–67.
56. Katzmarzyk PT. Physical activity, sedentary behavior, and health: paradigm paralysis or paradigm shift? Diabetes 2010;59:2717–25.
57. Yates T, Wilmot E, Khunti K, Biddle S, Gorely T, Davies M. Stand up for your health: is it time to rethink the physical activity paradigm? Diabetes Res Clin Pract 2011;93:292–4.
58. Pate RR, O'Neill JR, Lobelo F. The evolving definition of "sedentary". Exerc Sport Sci Rev 2008;36:173–8.

59. Wilmot E, Edwardson CL, Davies MJ, Gorely T, Gray L, Khunti K, et al. Sitting time in adults and the association with diabetes, cardiovascular disease and death: systematic review and meta-analysis. Diabetologia 2012;55:2895–2905.
60. Dunstan DW, Kingwell BA, Larsen R, et al. Breaking up prolonged sitting reduces postprandial glucose and insulin responses. Diabetes Care 2012;35:976–983.
61. Healy GN, Dunstan DW, Salmon J, Cerin E, Shaw JE, Zimmet PZ, et al. Breaks in sedentary time: beneficial associations with metabolic risk. Diabetes Care 2008;31:661–6.
62. Healy, GN, Dunstan DW, Salmon J, Shaw JE, Zimmet PZ, Owen N. Television time and continuous metabolic risk in physically active adults. Med Sci Sports Exerc 2008;40:639–45.
63. Sugiyama T, Healy GN, Dunstan DW, Salmon J, Owen N. Joint associations of multiple leisure-time sedentary behaviours and physical activity with obesity in Australian adults. Int J Behav Nutr Phys Act 2008;1:5:35.

CHAPTER 12

Overview: Potentials of new media for the training of health educators in the field of diabetes prevention

Daniel Tolks and Martin R. Fischer
Department of Medical Education, Munich University Hospital, Munich, Germany

Introduction

The successful breakthrough of digital technologies into nearly every private and public domain also entails changes for learning and teaching. According to the World Internet Usage [1], in 2011, 32.7% of the world's population had access to the internet, with a growth of 528.1% from the year 2000. North America shows the highest rate at 78.6%, and Africa the lowest rate with 13.5%. Nearly 61% of the population of Europe has internet access, with a growth rate of 376% between 2001 and 2011. Germany has the highest rate of internet use in Europe, with 65 million.

According to van Dyk [2, p.9], new media are characterized by three main aspects: media that are both integrated and interactive, and the use of digital code. New media include the internet, websites, computer multimedia, video games, CD-ROMs, and DVDs. New media do not include television programs, feature films, magazines, books, or paper-based publications unless they are delivered in digital form and have interactive elements included, for example e-books with comment features.

In the field of education, the integration of new media has not been completed. Conducting a search in PubMed and Google Scholar using the search terms "diabetes prevention"; "e-learning"; "new media"; "blended-learning";

Prevention of Diabetes, First Edition. Edited by Peter Schwarz and Prasuna Reddy.
© 2013 John Wiley & Sons, Ltd. Published 2013 by John Wiley & Sons, Ltd.

"Web 2.0"; "collaborative tools"; and "social web" resulted in only one article describing a health education program for diabetes experts in Thailand [3].

While research has been intensified, new technologies are being developed or are changing so rapidly that many more research questions emerge than can be addressed [4,5]. Furthermore, much of the hype surrounding e-learning has declined. Many expectations regarding the opportunities of new media for education have not been met so far [6–8]. Early voices demanding that traditional universities and schools be shut down are no longer heard. Gartner's hype cycles show that this is a common process for emerging technologies.

However, the boundaries between work and home, between formal and informal learning, between teachers and learners, between education and entertainment media, between content and learning management systems and Web 2.0 tools are blurred. In the Horizon Report 2012 [5] it was stated that people expect to be able to work, learn, and study whenever and wherever they want.

Today's online technologies can be used to immerse learners in cooperative ways, create learning communities, animate complex concepts, facilitate e-learning activities, involve learners in purposeful discussions, and offer learners an interactive online classroom that is a practical and effective alternative to traditional training environments [9]. Internet-based education permits learners to participate at a time and place convenient to them, facilitates instructional methods that might be difficult in other formats, and has the potential to tailor instruction to individual learner's needs. Internet-based learning has become an increasingly popular approach to medical education [10].

However, the idea of social learning software, especially in real educational scenarios, has not been widely developed, because too few innovators and early adopters are using social media technology to enhance existing curricula designs and learning behaviors. Often, the media literacy of educators lacks expertise and up-to-date experience. Educational opportunities to train the trainer in the field of media literacy are necessary. This is mostly provided by learning on the job and peer learning, but formal education also has an important role [11–13].

E-learning and the use of new media in the field of diabetes prevention can be used to inform, educate, or even target behavioral change in the general population or to assist training health facilitators, such as health personnel. Oomen-Early and Burke describe the challenges for the field: "Preparing health educators in today's technology-driven society requires faculty to adopt new teaching strategies which motivate and engage the Web 2.0 generation." [14, p.189].

There are a variety of activities using e-learning approaches and new media within the field of diabetes treatment, mostly to train patients [15,16]. These approaches cover e-learning platforms web-based information pages, and innovative projects like Serious Games.

Didactic concepts and e-learning approaches

A strict separation of didactic concepts and e-learning approaches is not possible because many of these concepts blend into each other.

E-learning
According to Hodson et al. [17], e-learning combines aspects of computer-based learning, interactive technologies, and computer-based distance-learning. E-learning activities use online technologies, such as chat rooms, discussion boards, email, or online classes to facilitate participation of e-learners in exercises related to the course and its e-learning objectives. Pure e-learning approaches have been replaced more and more by other didactic approaches. The term is still used as an overall description of the use of new technologies in education. In the field of health education, pure e-learning approaches are mostly used for continuing education because of widely disseminated target groups and the requirement for constant access. An example of e-learning is the ENeA project [18].

Blended learning
The term blended learning describes a hybrid learning concept. Blended learning combines face-to-face phases with e-learning phases of a learning environment to use the advantages of both settings for optimal knowledge acquisition [8]. Inherent in blended learning is a fundamental redesign of the instructional model, shifting from lecture to student-centered instruction, increasing all forms of interaction and incorporating assessment [19]. The blended learning approach is currently a widely used learning concept. Examples are the e-learning portal of the IMAGE project or the ICON learning platform [20,21].

Computer-based learning
Computer-based learning(CBL) refers to the use of computers as a key component of the educational environment. While this can refer to the

use of computers in a classroom, the term more broadly refers to a structured environment in which computers are used for teaching purposes. This definition is often used for multimedia learning software delivered on CD-ROM. The computer replaces the didactic components of education: imparting knowledge, offering provision and evaluation exercises [22].

Web-based learning

The term web-based learning emphasizes the fact that the user does not necessarily have to use a computer to use e-learning services. The learning takes place on the web, independent of the technology that is used to access the web. Video or handheld consoles can be used to access the web. This term is used more often than CBL.

Online case-based learning

A case describes an "actual situation, commonly involving a decision, challenge, opportunity, problem, or an issue faced by a person (or persons) in an organization" [22]. Most authors describe case-based learning (CBL) as an active self-directed enquiry into situations containing a number of domain-related issues [23]. Online case-based learning provides students with an environment to interact with a case in diversified ways and settings. Furthermore, instructional multimedia components can help students gain a richer comprehension of the concepts and principles surrounding the case [24].

Mobile learning

Mobile learning uses cell phones, smartphones, portable media players, and other portable devices. According to the Pewinternet.org [25], in May 2011 two in five cell phone owners (42%) in the United States owned a smartphone. Since 83% of Americans own some kind of mobile phone, this means that one-third of all American adults (35%) are smartphone owners. The 2011 Horizon Report stated that internet-capable mobile devices will outnumber computers within the next year. This is enabled by the convergence of the growing number of internet-capable mobile devices, the increasingly flexile web content, and continued development of the networks that support connectivity. Mobiles enable access to information, social networks, and tools for learning [26]. The biggest advantage is that learning can take place almost everywhere and at any time. The convergence of several technologies on mobile devices, such as annotation tools, applications for creative and social networking tools and the potential for education means this is already being demonstrated in hundreds of projects at higher education institutions [26].

Digital game-based learning and Serious Games

There is much discussion about a definition of the term game-based learning, or Serious Games. Sawyer and Smith [27] offer the following definition: "Any computerized game whose chief mission is not entertainment and all entertainment games which can be reapplied to a different mission other than entertainment."

Nearly 8% of all Serious Games have been developed for health-related topics. According to a literature review [28], 24 of 25 Serious Games for health demonstrated a broad spectrum of desirable outcomes from knowledge increases, attitude, behavior, and other health-related changes. These games are able to foster collaboration, problem-solving, and procedural thinking [5].

There has been an early approach to use Serious Games for the treatment of diabetes in children. The game *Packy and Marlon* was developed by Click Health. Studies showed that there has been a positive effect concerning aspects of higher perceived self-efficacy for diabetes self-management, increasing the patient's communication with their parents about diabetes, improving their daily diabetes self-management behaviors, and a 77% reduction in diabetes-related emergencies [29]. According to the Horizon Report 2012 [5], game-based learning is one of the most important technologies in the field of education in the future.

Web 2.0 and social software

The term Web 2.0 and social software encompasses a variety of different meanings that include an increased emphasis on user-generated content, data and content sharing and collaborative effort, together with the use of various kinds of applications, new ways of interacting with web-based applications, and the use of the web as a platform for generating, re-purposing, and consuming content. Because of their ease of use and rapidity of deployment, Web 2.0 applications offer the opportunity for fast information sharing and ease of collaboration [30]. The terms Web 2.0, social software, social media, and e-learning 2.0 are often used synonymously.

According to Schmidt [31, p. 32]: "Social software refers to those online-based applications and services that facilitate information management, identity management, and relationship management by providing (partial) publics of hyper textual and social networks." According to Kaplan and Haenlein [32, p. 61] social software is: "a group of Internet-based applications that build on the ideological and technological foundations of Web 2.0, and that allow the creation and exchange of user-generated content."

Downes [33] pointed out that the term Web 2.0 describes not a technology but rather an idea of cooperation and networks. Wilson et al. [34, p. 2] gave the following definition: "Web 2.0 refers to the second generation of the Web, wherein interoperable, user-centered web applications and services promote social connectedness, media and information sharing, user-created content, and collaboration among individuals and organizations."

The term social software is often used as a summary of applications that promote the collaborative assembling and working on content, like wikis or blogs. A way to explain the new aspects of Web 2.0 applications is to compare them to the "old Web 1.0". In "Web 1.0," few authors provided content such as communication and course management tools, from web page to course management systems, PowerPoint presentations, email, bulletin boards, and chat rooms. Web 1.0 put the learner in the center of the teaching method, improved the learning experience, facilitated student–faculty and student–student communication for a wide audience of relatively passive readers. In Web 2.0, users use the web as a platform to generate, re-purpose, and consume shared content. The web also becomes a platform for social software that enables groups of users to socialize and work together in a collaborative way. This change of use is largely based on existing web data, sharing mechanisms being used to share content and get in contact with other users [35]. Web 2.0 is not the counterpart of the "classic" Web 1.0 but rather a further development of it [36]. According to Alby [37], the further development and change in technologies has also influenced the frameworks of the web. Without low priced broadband internet, experienced users, open-source software, and easy-to-use applications, the World Wide Web (www) would not have evolved in this way. McFedries [38] identifies the main characteristics of the Web 2.0 movement, highlighting the social perspective of relation, collaboration, and user-participated architecture:

- Content is user-created and maintained;
- User-created and maintained content requires radical trust;
- Application usability allows rich user experience;
- Combining data from different sources leads to creation of new services; and

- Services get better as the number of users increases in architecture of participation.

The application of social software in learning environments offers a learning-oriented educational approach and can promote a cooperative and self-organized learning process. Web 2.0 applications are suitable for the constructivism learning approach [39]. When applied in education, Web 2.0 technology entails some fundamental shifts in teaching and learning. Conole and Alevizou [40] point out that Web 2.0 practice encourages crossing traditional disciplinary boundaries of knowledge (i.e., knowledge can be personalized and re-appropriated), and in collaborative inquiry and knowledge production there are greater opportunities for access, debate, and transparency.

There are further developments such as Web 3.0 or semantic web that was described by the World Wide Web Consortium (W3C) and defined by Berners-Lee as "a web of data that can be processed directly and indirectly by machines" [41]. The Semantic Web provides a common framework that allows data to be shared and reused across applications, enterprises, and community boundaries. This emerging technology and its opportunities will not be covered in this chapter.

Overview of Web 2.0 applications

There is a large variety in Web 2.0 technology. We illustrate the most common applications in the field of education. Mostly, Web 2.0 technology is not used alone but rather implemented with other applications (e.g., social networks containing other applications).

Blogs

The term blog is a contraction of "web log" and describes a virtual multi-media log or online diary used to share information and opinions of the user [37]. Blogs are simple content management tools enabling non-experts to display (post) information, articles, or share his/her opinions on different topics, while readers can comment by post or enter into a discussion with the author or other readers. They are published chronologically, with links and commentary on various issues of interest. Blogs are networked between several users who post thoughts that often focus upon a common theme. Engaging people with knowledge sharing, reflection, and debate, they often attract a large and dedicated readership [30]. There has been a shift from blogs containing personal information to those offering more professional information. Online journals existed before the invention of blogs, but the widely distributed and easy-to-use software offered everyone the opportunity to use blogs.

The implementation of blogs in an educational framework offers the participants of a course the opportunity to share their thoughts and promotes peer-to-peer discussions to reflect critically on their own thoughts. The application of blogs in curricula was already tested in studies finding positive effects regarding the motivation, interaction within the team, critical thinking, and an overall higher course satisfaction [14,42–45]. Furthermore, the constructivist learning approach of blogging may help increase a learner's research, evaluation, technology practice, and media literacy. Consistent with online learning, blogs provide both learners and instructors with a high level of autonomy [14,46].

Examples of educational implementation of blogs:

- A group using their own blog can build up a corpus on interrelated knowledge via posts and comments in a course; and
- The course moderator can use the blog to inform the course participants about the newest topics in the field of diabetes prevention and course-related information as well.

Wikis

A wiki (*wiki* is Hawaiian for "swift") is a web-based application that offers the user the opportunity to work together to create new content based on the wisdom of the group. Wiki features includes easy editing, versioning capabilities, and article discussions. The very process of collaboration leads to a Darwinian type of "survival of the fittest" content within a web page. The veracity of these resources can be assured through careful monitoring, moderation, and feedback [30]. The system offers the opportunity to build a corpus of knowledge in a process of creating, editing, and discussion [35]. The most prominent example of a wiki is Wikipedia. However, the general quality and scientific background is sometimes lacking and inconsistent.

According to Döbeli Honegger [47], the application of wikis in an educational framework is relatively easy, though some preconditions must be set up for its successful implementation: a technical prerequisite, a tutorial for users, clear work instructions and an implemented moderation.

There are other collaborative editing tools that allow users in different locations to edit the same document at the same time. Examples are Google Docs and Spreadsheets. These technologies can be implemented into a course curriculum to foster collaboration between the course participants.

Examples of educational implementation of wikis:

- In a health-related online curriculum users could use a wiki for the production of collaboratively edited material.
- Wikis can be used for an annotated reading list of one or more course teachers.
- Wikis can be used as a class project to foster the incremental accretion of knowledge by a group or production of collaboratively edited material and group work projects.
- Wikis can be used as a feedback tool by a teacher. They can give feedback during the process of group work if they also have access to the documents being edited by the group in order to moderate the learning and creation process.
- Course participants can use the wiki to give feedback to other group members.
- Wikis can also be used as a part of a virtual community of practice

Podcasts

The term podcast (a blend of the words iPod and broadcast) describes time and location independent digital audio or video files. Free software enables computer users to subscribe to regular podcast feeds (audio/video RSS feeds), download them automatically, and watch or listen to them on a portable device such as an MP3/MP4 player or any laptop or desktop computer [48]. Podcasting is a way in which the listener may keep up with recent audio or video content. Most podcasts or videocasts are filmed face-to-face lectures and generally lacking didactic and pedagogic principles of media use [49].

Examples of educational implementation of podcasts:

- Podcasts can be used to provide material in the pre- and post-assignment phase of a curriculum or record lectures conducted in face-to-face phases to allow course participants to learn from lectures in their own time.
- Podcasts can be used to provide course-related information as part of a pre-assessment.
- Podcasts can also be used to share lectures and conference talks as a part of the learning materials.

Social networking

Based on the principle of Milgram's small world paradigm, social networking services are online group-forming applications that connect people through shared information interests and allow them to manage their interactions with others on a massive scale [48,50].

These networks (e.g., Facebook, MySpace) collect data about members and store the information as user profiles which are shared among site members. Social networking services enable users to share information within a shifting network of colleagues through user profiles linking users to others posting similar information [48]. Some social networking services combine or bundle several Web 2.0 features together (instant messaging, social bookmarking, blogs, and podcasts). However, many commercial online social networks have issues concerning the protection of data and privacy.

Examples of educational implementation of social networking:

- The networks can be used to disseminate and discuss questions in a network of experts.
- Social networks can be used at a professional level for group learning.
- Social networks can be used to maintain a network of health educators formerly gathered together within a course curriculum like the diabetes prevention manager curriculum.

Syndication and notification technologies

A feed reader can be used to centralize all the recent changes in the sources of interest and the user can easily access this information directly, as a list or as a summary. The most prominent notification is an RSS (Really Simple Syndication). In an e-learning curriculum where a wiki or a discussion forum is used, the participants can be informed about recent changes, new entries, or new learning content.

Special search features and social search engines

A similar concept is adopted by this application which can be thought of as a community-powered search engine, tailored to produce only the targeted search results that the search engine owner/creator and her/his community want. The search results from a social search engines are potentially more relevant than those produced by general search engines, as they represent focused, targeted web views, based on the search behavior and search patterns of the associated community of users. An example is Swicki, which is a diabetes-related social search engine.

Media-sharing services

These systems store user-contributed media and make it available for every user of the web. Examples are YouTube (movies), iTunes (podcasts and vidcasts), Flickr (photos), and Slideshare (presentations). These media-sharing services can be used to improve the course curriculum using educational videos and multimedia applications to foster the learning outcomes of a course curriculum.

New media in diabetes prevention

Benefits of the use of e-learning and new media for the training of health educators

Benefits of e-learning approaches are the time flexibility regarding the learning processes, the constant availability of learning content, the variety of different learning resources, the diversity of learning and teaching approaches, as well as the creation of new social contexts and different collaboration tools, such as the use of online discussion forums. The use of learning media promotes the learning experience as well as the personal engagement of the course participants. Every learning medium has to be tested for didactic usefulness within the framework of the learning environment.

According to Boulos et al. [30], wikis, blogs, and podcasts could offer a way to enhance the learning experience, and deepen levels of learners' engagement and collaboration within the digital learning environments. Media such as online discussion forums and the use of blogs assist peer-to-peer discussion and promote new collaborative work, which is crucial for a successful learning process. Paton et al. [51] conducted a review of the literature about the use of social media tools in medical and health education and found little empirical evidence to support the use of social media tools in medical and health education. They pointed out that social media are a rapidly evolving range of tools, websites, and online experiences and it is likely that the topic is too broad to draw definitive conclusions from any particular study but nonetheless recommend the use of social media.

Furthermore, the media literacy of each participant will be improved by using new media. By using the new media, participants will learn how to use this technology effectively for health promotion activities. Preparing health educators in today's technology-driven society requires the faculty to adopt new teaching strategies to motivate and engage Web 2.0 generation.

Projects in the field of diabetes prevention using new media

The only project that was found by conducting a search in PubMed and Google Scholar using the words "diabetes prevention"; "e-learning"; "new media"; "blended-learning"; "Web 2.0"; "collaborative tools"; and "social web" was a health education program for diabetes experts in Thailand [3]. This project was a tailored diabetes prevention education program conducted by the University of Waterloo, Canada, and the Institute of Nutrition, Mahidol University, Thailand. A blended learning approach using a learning management system, classroom sections and providing CD-ROMs was conducted. Online materials including videotaped lectures, Youtube videos, readings, monthly newsletters, and community resources have been used [3].

Despite the search on PubMed and Google Scholar, there are only a few diabetes prevention projects using new media. These projects took place in Germany.

An example for using a blended learning approach is the e-learning portal of the IMAGE project to train diabetes type 2 prevention managers. The e-learning portal is implemented within the framework of a blended learning approach to train diabetes type 2 prevention managers. The portal offers tools for collaborative work like a discussion forum and the possibility to use wikis and blogs to foster the collaborative learning of the course participants.

The e-learning portal, Das Präventionsnetzwerk, developed by the group of Peter Schwartz at the University of Dresden based on the IMAGE curriculum is also available to be used as a training tool for the education of diabetes prevention experts. There are many activities in the field of diabetes prevention using e-learning platforms such as the KoQuaP of the German Diabetes Foundation. The KoQuaP offers evaluation of diabetes prevention activities based on an e-learning approach using a learning management platform (Table 12.1).

New media in health communication and its potential for diabetes prevention

The focus of this chapter is to give an overview of the potentials of Web 2.0 applications to foster the learning processes and outcomes in the training of health experts and personnel. The use of new media can also be used as a tool for media-based health communication. This includes a variety of different scenarios and would fill a whole new chapter. We give a brief overview of this field. Social networks can be used as self-support groups or patient networks as well as promotion platforms in the field of diabetes prevention. Blogs and wikis may be used to share health-related information. There is a great variety of possibilities for communicating diabetes-related topics and even tailored information can be provided. The

Table 12.1 Use of new media in diabetes prevention.

Name	Purpose	Didactic concept	Use of technology	Link
IMAGE	Training of diabetes type 2 prevention managers	Blended learning	Learn Management System (LMS), wikis, blogs, discussion forum	www.image-project.eu
Sranacharoenpong et al.	Training of health workers in the field of diabetes prevention	Blended learning	Learn Management System (LMS)	No website
Das Präventionsnetzwerk	Training of diabetes type 2 prevention managers	Blended learning	Learn Management System (LMS), discussion forum	http://nebel. tumainiserver.de/ tumaini/index.php
KoQuaP	Quality management and evaluation	E-learning	Learn Management System (LMS), discussion forum	www.koquap.de

Centers for Disease and Prevention (CDC) for instance offers tailored information that will be sent to mobile phone of the user [52] and uses Facebook, Twitter, and other new Web 2.0 applications to inform the general population about health-related topics. The German Diabetes Federation (Deutsche Diabetes Stiftung) uses Facebook to share the newest trends and scientific articles and start discussions with users. Other health communication strategies like Entertainment-Education and the use of Serious Games can be used to communicate health-related topics and target health behavior for high risk groups in the field of diabetes [53,54]. The study of Thompson et al. [55] showed that video games, enhanced by behavior-change technology and motivating stories, offer opportunities to promote diet and physical change for diabetes and obesity prevention.

In the field of health communication, a blog is also a good way to offer health information to the general population or to risk groups. . Furthermore, blogging may encourage individuals to take social and political action outside of the virtual environment.

Wikis can be used to share health-related information with the general population or high-risk groups developed by diabetes experts and patients.

The benefit of such cooperation would be the more prominent perspective of patients to related issues of diabetes. Online social networking services are often used for support and self-help groups to connect people with the same issues. In the field of diabetes, an example is the MySpace CURE DiABETES group (http://groups.myspace.com/cureDiABETES) organized by patients and supporters. Podcasts can also be used to share health-related information with the general population and to provide useful information for risk groups. A feed can also be used by people in a risk group to get the latest information about health-related topics. Facilitators have direct access to the risk group and can very easily and quickly provide relevant information for the target group.

Conclusions

Not since the invention of the web and its subsequent development as a multimedia platform have we seen such an exciting array of emerging technologies, yet to date relatively few health care organizations have taken up the tools and strategic advantages offered by Web 2.0. Most of these activities and projects using e-learning approaches and new media take place within the field of diabetes treatment but only a few projects are using these approaches for diabetes prevention.

According to the results of Cook et al. [10], nearly all no-intervention comparison studies found a benefit; a wide variety of internet-based interventions can be used effectively in medical education. Despite the fact that many studies have already found positive results concerning the effectiveness of the use of e-learning approaches and new media to educate and train, only a few projects are visible to the scientific community. There may be more projects using these learning approaches, but the literature review showed only a few projects using these features. The reason is that even institutions that are eager to use these new technologies are limited by human and financial resources as well as having a lack of expertise and experience [5].

Outlook

The potential of Web 2.0 applications can foster the training of health experts and personnel and can also be used to inform, raise awareness, and target health behavior change in the general population. New technologies offer vast opportunities to promote learning in the field of training health experts like the prevention manager. However, the movers and shakers within the field of diabetes prevention should carefully verify the use of Web 2.0 applications for their projects.

Future trends should be closely monitored to prevent developing technologies no longer used in a fast-changing digital society and to develop strategies to use the state of the art technologies that enhance learning and education.

We would like to encourage all health educators to take advantage of the opportunity to use new technology with all its possible benefits to improve the training of health experts and health communication in the future. Or, in the words of William Gibson in the presentation of O'Reilly: "The future is here. It's just not evenly distributed yet."

References

1. World Internet Usage Statistics News and Population Stats. 2012. Available from: www.internetworldstats.com/stats.htm (accessed 9 March 2013).
2. van Dijk J. The Network Society: Social aspects of new media. SAGE; 2006.
3. Sranacharoenpong K, Hanning RM, Sirichakwal PP, Chittchang U. Process and outcome evaluation of a diabetes prevention education program for community healthcare workers in Thailand. Educ Health (Abingdon) 2009;22(3):335.
4. Fischer F, Mandl H, Todorova A. Lehren und Lernen mit neuen Medien. In: Tippelt R, Schmidt B, Herausgeber. Handbuch Bildungsforschung. Wiesbaden: VS Verlag für Sozialwissenschaften; 2012: pp. 753–71. Available from: www.springerlink.com/content/v787xq10401g3g53/ (accessed 9 March 2013).
5. Johnson L, Adams S, Cummins M. The NMC Horizon Report: 2012 Higher Education Edition. Austin, Texas: The New Media Consortium; 2012.
6. Dittler U. Einführung–E-Learning in der betrieblichen Aus-und Weiterbildung. Dittler, Ullrich. E-Learning–Einsatzkonzepte und Erfolgsfaktoren des Lernens mit interaktiven Medien. München/Wien; Oldenbourg Wissenschaftsverlag: 2003; pp. 9–22.
7. Mathes M. E-Learning in der Hochschullehre: Überholt Technik Gesellschaft? Medienpädagogik-Onlinezeitschrift, Hrsg.: B. Bachmair, C. de Witt, P. Diepold, K. Ernst, H. Moser, D. Süss, Zürich. 2002. Available from: www. medienpaed. com/02-1/mathes1. pdf (accessed 9 March 2013).
8. Mandl H, Kopp B. Blended Learning: Forschungsfragen und Perspektiven. 2006.
9. Watkins R. 75 e-learning activities: making online learning interactive. Pfeiffer; 2005.
10. Cook DA, Levinson AJ, Garside S, Dupras DM, Erwin PJ, Montori VM. Internet-based learning in the health professions: a meta-analysis. JAMA 2008;300(10):1181.
11. Kerres M, Euler D, Seufert S, Hasanbegovic J, Voss B. Lehrkompetenz für eLearning-Innovationen in der Hochschule: Ergebnisse einer explorativen Studie zu Massnahmen der Entwicklung von eLehrkompetenz. 2005.

12. Bremer C. Fit fürs Web 2.0? Ein Medienkompetenzzertifikat für zukünftige Lehrer/innen. Offener Bildungsraum Hochschule. Münster: Waxmann; 2008: pp. 134–46.

13. Erpenbeck J, Sauter W. Kompetenzentwicklung im Netz. New Blended Learning mit Web 2.0. Köln: Kluwer; 2007.

14. Oomen-Early J, Burke S. Entering the blogosphere: blogs as teaching and learning tools in health education. Int Electr J Health Educ 2007;10:11.

15. Chomutare T, Fernandez-Luque L, Arsand E, Hartvigsen G. Features of mobile diabetes applications: review of the literature and analysis of current applications compared against evidence-based guidelines. J Med Internet Res 2011;13(3):e65.

16. Nordqvist C, Hanberger L, Timpka T, Nordfeldt S. Health professionals' attitudes towards using a Web 2.0 portal for child and adolescent diabetes care: qualitative study. J Med Internet Res 2009;11(2):e12.

17. Hodson P, Connolly M, Saunders D. Can computer-based learning support adult learners? J Further Higher Educ 2001;25(3):325–35.

18. Early Nutrition Academy – Early Nutrition eAcademy (ENeA). Available from: www.early-nutrition.org/enea.html (accessed 9 March 2013).

19. Graham CR, Dziuban C. Blended learning environments. In: Spector JM, Merrill MD, van Merrienboer J, Driscoll MP, eds. Handbook of Research on Educational Communications and Technology, 3rd edn. 2008; pp. 269–76.

20. Tolks D, Gruhl U, Puhl S, Fischer M. Entwicklungen und Einführung eines E-Health Portals im Rahmen des IMAGE-Projekts: Typ 2 Diabetes-Prävention in Europa. e-Health 2010 Informationstechnologien und Telematik im Gesundheitswesen. 1. Aufl. medical future verlag; 2009: pp. 288–92.

21. Tolks D, Quattrochi J, Fischer MR. Internationales kooperatives Lernen mit der fallbasierten Lernumgebung ICON. E-Health 2011. Solingen: Medical Future Verlag; 2010L pp. 284–8.

22. Dittler U. E-Learning: Einsatzkonzepte und Erfolgsfaktoren des Lernens mit interaktiven Medien. 2, überarb. und erg. Aufl. München; Wien; Oldenbourg; 2003.

23. Andrews L. Preparing General Education Pre-Service Teachers for Inclusion: Web-Enhanced Case-Based Instruction. J Spec Educ Technol 2002;17(3):27–35.

24. Lee S, Lee J, Liu X, Bonk CJ, Magjuka RJ. A review of case-based learning practices in an online MBA program: a program-level case study. Educ Technol Soc 2009; 12:178–90.

25. Pew Internet. How smartphone owners describe their phones. Pew Research Center's Internet and American Life Project. Available from: www.pewinternet.org/Infographics/2011/Smartphones.aspx (accessed 9 March 2013).

26. Johnson L, Smith R, Willis H, Levine A, Haywood K. The 2011 Horizon Report. Austin, Texas: The New Media Consortium; 2011.

27. Sawyer B, Smith P. Serious Games Taxonomy. 2008.

28. Baranowski T, Buday R, Thompson D, Baranowski J. Playing for real: video games and stories for health-related behavior change. Am J Prevent Med 2008;34(1):74–82.

29. Brown SJ, Lieberman DA, Germeny BA, Fan YC, Wilson DM, Pasta DJ. Educational video game for juvenile diabetes: results of a controlled trial. Med Inform (Lond). 1997;22(1):77–89.

30. Boulos M, Maramba I, Wheeler S. Wikis, blogs and podcasts: a new generation of Web-based tools for virtual collaborative clinical practice and education. BMC Med Educ 2006;6(1):41.

31. Schmidt J. Social Software. Onlinegestütztes Informations-, Identitäts-und Beziehungsmanagement. Forschungsjournal Neue Soziale Bewegungen. 2006;19(2): 37–47.

32. Kaplan AM, Haenlein M. Users of the world, unite! The challenges and opportunities of Social Media. Business Horizons 2010;53(1):59–68.

33. Downes S. E-learning 2.0. eLearn Magazine. 2005;2005(10).

34. Wilson DW, Lin X, Longstreet P, Sarker S. Web 2.0: A definition, literature review, and directions for future research. AMCIS 2011 Proceedings. 2011. Available from: http://aisel.aisnet.org/amcis2011_submissions/368/ (accessed 9 March 2013).

35. Franklin T, van Harmelen M. Web 2.0 for content for learning and teaching in higher education. 2007. Available from: http://www.jisc.ac.uk/media/documents/ programmes/digitalrepositories/web2-content-learning-and-teaching.pdf (accessed 9 March 2013).

36. Schiefner M, Kerres M. Web 2.0 in der Hochschullehre. E-Learning: Einsatzkonzepte und Erfolgsfaktoren des Lernens mit interaktiven Medien. München: Oldenburg; 2011.

37. Alby T. Web 2.0: Konzepte, Anwendungen, Technologien. Hanser Verlag; 2008.

38. McFedries P. Technically speaking the web, take two. Spectrum, IEEE. 2006;43(6):68.

39. Jadin T. Social Software für kollaboratives Lernen. E-Learning, digitale Medien und lebenslanges Lernen: Schriftenreihe E-Learning. Linz: Trauner. 2007;23–35.

40. Conole G, Alevizou P. A literature review of the use of Web 2.0 tools in Higher Education. Milton Keynes, UK: The Open University. Available from: www. heacademy.ac.uk/assets/EvidenceNEt/Conole_Alevizou_2010.pdf (accessed 9 March 2013).

41. W3C Semantic Web Activity. Available from: www.w3.org/2001/sw/ (accessed 9 March 2013).

42. Beldarrain Y. Distance education trends: Integrating new technologies to foster student interaction and collaboration. Distance Educ 2006;27(2):139–53.

43. Halavais A, Hernández-Ramos P. Blogs, threaded discussions accentuate constructivist teaching. Online Classroom 2004;1.

44. Williams JB, Jacobs J. Exploring the use of blogs as learning spaces in the higher education sector. Australas J Educat Technol 2004;20(2):232–47.

45. Oravec JA. Bookmarking the world: Weblog applications in education. J Adolesc Adult Literacy 2002;45(7):616–21.

46. Süss D, Lampert C, Wijnen CW. Medienpädagogik: Ein Studienbuch zur Einführung. 1. Aufl. Wiesbaden: VS Verlag; 2009.

47. Döbeli Honegger B. Wiki und die starken Texte–Schreibprojekte mit Wikis. Deutschmagazin 2006;1(06):15–9.

48. Boulos MN, Wheeler S. The emerging Web 2.0 social software: an enabling suite of sociable technologies in health and health care education. Health Info Libr J 2007;24(1):2–23.

49. Stöber A, Göcks M. Die unberechtigte Angst vor der Konserve: Machen Vorlesungsaufzeichnungen und Podcasts die Präsenzlehre überflüssig. E-Learning: Eine Zwischenbilanz. Kritischer Rückblick als Basis eines Aufbruchs. Münster: Waxmann; 2009: pp. 117–32.

50. Travers J, Milgram S. An experimental study of the small world problem. Sociometry 1969;32:425–43.

51. Paton C, Bamidis P, Eysenbach G, Hansen M, Cabrer M. Experience in the use of social medial in medical and health education. IMIA Yearbook 2011;2011:61.
52. CDC – Learn More. Available from: www.cdc.gov/mobile/textmessaging/ (accessed 9 March 2013).
53. Singhal A, Cody M, Rogers E, Sabido M. Entertainment-Education and Social Change: History, Research, and Practice. Mahwah, NJ: Lawrence Erlbaum; 2003.
54. Lampert C, Schwinge C, Tolks D. Der gespielte Ernst des Lebens: Bestandsaufnahme und Potenziale von Serious Games (for Health). Medien Pädagogik. 2009. Available from: www.medienpaed.com/zs/content/view/220/67/ (accessed 9 March 2013).
55. Thompson D, Baranowski T, Buday R, Baranowski J, Juliano M, Frazior MK. In pursuit of change: youth response to intensive goal setting embedded in a serious video game. J Diabetes Sci Technol 2007;1(6):907–17.

CHAPTER 13

Practical approach to the implementation of diabetes prevention

Avivit Cahn[1,2], Itamar Raz[2] and Baruch Itzhak[3]

[1] Endocrinology and Metabolism Service, Department of Medicine, Hadassah-Hebrew University Medical Center, Jerusalem, Israel
[2] The Diabetes Unit, Department of Medicine, Hadassah-Hebrew University Medical Center, Jerusalem, Israel
[3] Israel National Diabetes Prevention Committee, Jerusalem, Israel

The modern era of obesity and physical inactivity has led to an immense increase in the prevalence of chronic noncommunicable diseases, in particular the metabolic syndrome and diabetes mellitus and its complications. In the last decade, much effort has been directed at diabetes prevention and lifestyle modification. Observational studies, as well as randomized controlled trials targeting main modifiable risk factors for diabetes in high-risk populations, demonstrated a risk reduction of up to 58% by diet and exercise, and 25–30% by pharmacologic treatment [1–3]. Nationwide programs have been established in several countries in an effort to translate data from interventional studies to real-life settings [4–6]. Economic evaluation verified that programs aimed at primary prevention of type 2 diabetes are cost effective [7].

In this chapter we describe the programs developed in Israel for the prevention of diabetes. The programs are directed at two levels:

1. *High-risk populations:* screening high-risk populations for undiagnosed diabetes and prediabetes, and interventions directed at diabetes prevention.
2. *Whole population:* programs directed at the entire population, encouraging adaptation of a healthier lifestyle.

Epidemiology

Currently, it is estimated that the diabetic population in Israel includes approximately 500 000 people with type 1 and type 2 diabetes. This estimate consists of approximately 60% of diagnosed patients treated with medications, 25% of treatment-naïve patients, and 15% of undiagnosed patients. An additional 500 000 people are estimated to have prediabetes [8–10].

Obesity has become a worldwide epidemic expanding at an alarming rate. The Israeli National Health Survey of 2008 found over 30% of the adult population was overweight and 15% was obese [9].

A recent survey in kindergarten children in central Israel found 15% of the children to be overweight [11]. A survey conducted in 2003–2004 among children in grades 7–12 found 7.4% of the boys and 3.9% of the girls were obese [12]. Among 17-year-old Israeli conscripts, the prevalence of overweight was 4.1% in males and 3.3% in females; an additional 12% were borderline overweight [13]. The increased rates of overweight in these young age groups indicates the emergence of an obesity epidemic in Israel.

Combining forces

In Israel, the National Health Insurance Law, enacted in 1994, required that all citizens be registered in one of four health plans: Clalit, Maccabi, Meuchedet or Leumit. The health plans are obligated to provide preventive, ambulatory, and inpatient care for their members [14]. The shift between the health plans is minimal (1–1.5% per year) [15]; thus, they have an incentive to invest in preventive medicine.

The National Council of Diabetes, which was founded in 2005, consults with the Director General of the Ministry of Health on professional policy issues related to prevention, care, and therapy for diabetes in Israel. This council was nominated by the Director General and is comprised of representatives from each of the four health plans, leading physicians in the field of diabetes and its related complications, paramedical experts, epidemiologists, and representatives from the Israel Diabetes Association and the Juvenile Diabetes Association. In order to deal with the diabetes and obesity epidemic in Israel, the Ministry of Health and the National Council of Diabetes formulated a nationwide program aimed at lifestyle modification of the population at large, as well as that of specific population groups. The operational principles include:

1. Joint operation by the Ministries of Health, Education, and Culture and Sports.
2. Operation of programs modeled on similar plans implemented worldwide and proven as cost-effective.
3. Establishment of cooperation between governmental and private bodies with pooling of resources.
4. Ongoing monitoring and evaluation throughout each program.

The programs are aimed at both decreasing the risk of progression to diabetes for high-risk populations with prediabetes, and at increasing health awareness in the general population.

Screening and treating prediabetes

The purpose of diagnosing prediabetes is to identify the segment of the population at increased risk for the development of both diabetes and cardiovascular disease (CVD) so that interventions (lifestyle and pharmacologic) can be initiated.

Currently, patients who are diagnosed with impaired fasting glucose are identified and counseled by their family doctor and referred to a dietitian.

In 2008, the National Council of Diabetes presented a plan, targeting high-risk populations, in order to prevent their progression to diabetes. The program is to be initiated during the year 2013 and comprises of four steps:

1. *Identifying high-risk populations:*
   - Advertisement to the general public – with the slogan of "Before sweet turns bitter" appealing to those at high risk to have their fasting glucose checked. Advertisements will run for 1 year using television, radio, and newspaper media.
   - Family doctors will be alerted to recognize their high-risk patients and call them to come and test for fasting blood glucose. High-risk patients are defined as those fulfilling one of the following criteria:
     - Age >40 years
     - Body mass index (BMI) >25 with one additional risk factor of the following:
       1. Hypertension – blood pressure >140/90 mmHg;
       2. High-density lipoprotein (HDL) <35 mg/dL;
       3. Triglycerides >200 mg/dL;
       4. Ethnicity: Arab or Ethiopian;

5. History of gestational diabetes mellitus or of delivery of baby >4 kg;
6. History of CVD;
7. Polycystic ovary syndrome; or
8. Ingestion of medications that may cause glucose intolerance.

2. *Screening:*
   - Medical history – demographics, family history of diabetes;
   - Anthropometric measurements – height, weight, blood pressure, waist circumference; and
   - Fasting blood glucose, HbA1c, and lipid profile.

3. *Risk assessment.* Risk assessment is calculated according to Table 13.1, dependent upon family history of diabetes, BMI, age, triglyceride level, and fasting plasma glucose. Table 13.1 is derived from the follow-up data of Israeli men aged 26–45 for up to 12 years [16]. Those in whom the risk for progression to diabetes is calculated to be over 10% in the upcoming 6 years will comprise the intervention group.

4. *Intervention and monitoring.* Patients with fasting glucose of >126 mg/dL will undergo repeat testing to verify the diagnosis of diabetes. If confirmed, they will be treated according to international guidelines.

Patients with less than a 10% risk of progression to diabetes in the coming 6 years will be referred for testing every 3 years. The intervention group will comprise those with an increased risk (>10%) of progressing to overt diabetes in the coming 6 years. The intervention will focus on lifestyle modification with predefined targets, including:

- Weight loss of 5–7% in those who are overweight or obese;
- Reduction of the fat content of calories to less than 30% and saturated fat to less than 10%;
- Increased intake of dietary fiber; and
- 150 minutes of exercise per week.

Patients in the intervention group will be referred for six sessions delivered by a multidisciplinary team, including physicians, nurses, physiotherapists or physical educators, dietitians, and psychologists or social workers. All members of the team will undergo specific training for conducting the sessions. The following topics should be discussed:

- Complications of obesity, diabetes, and the metabolic syndrome;
- The components of a healthy diet;
- Suggested exercise regimes, suitable for a heterogeneous population;
- Barriers to adherence and ways to overcome them; and
- Creating a healthy environment at work and at home.

Table 13.1 Six year risk of developing diabetes according to data from the Israeli Diabetes Research Group (16). The shaded areas indicate increased risk (>10%) for developing diabetes.

Family history	BMI	Age	Triglycerides	Fasting plasma glucose				
				<80	81–90	91–99	100–109	110–125
No	<25	<45	<150	<1	<1	<1	1.5	6
			≥150	<1	<1	2	3	10
	25–30	<30	<150	<1	<1	<1	2	5
			≥150	<1	1	3	4	10
		30–45	<150	<1	1.5	2	2.5	14
			≥150	1	2	3	5	18
	≥30	<30	<150	0	<1	3	5	6
			≥150	0	2	3	10	12
		30–45	<150	0	2.5	3	6	15
			≥150	0	2.5	4	9	25
Yes	<25	<45	<150	<1	<1	1	3	11
			≥150	<1	<1	4	5	15
	25–30	<30	<150	<1	<1	1	4	12
			≥150	<1	1	3	6	15
		30–45	<150	2	2	3	6	20
			≥150	3	4	6	10	30
	≥30	<30	<150	0	<1	3	8	40
			≥150	0	2	5	15	50
		30–45	<150	0	2	5	10	40
			≥150	0	5	10	30	50

The sessions are held at local clinics, both in the morning and in the evenings, to enable as many people as possible to attend. The first five sessions last 2 hours each, every other week. The sixth session is held 3 months later to encourage long-term adherence to lifestyle modification.

Fasting blood glucose testing is repeated every 6 months. In cases of persistent impaired fasting glucose (IFG) levels for over a year, a glucose tolerance test may be performed to diagnose impaired glucose tolerance (IGT). In those patients with both IFG and IGT, treatment with metformin may be considered in any of the following conditions:

- Age <60 years;
- BMI >35;

- First-degree relative with type 2 diabetes
- Triglycerides >150;
- HDL <35 mg/dL
- Hypertension – defined as BP >140/90 mmHg or taking antihypertensive medication; and
- HbA1c >6 mg%.

Medical treatment with acarbose or orlistat may also be considered. Bariatric surgery should be considered according to guidelines. The intervention program is accompanied by ongoing monitoring to evaluate its efficacy.

National programs targeted at the obesity epidemic

In order to avert the upcoming obesity epidemic and the risks that accompany it, an interministerial action team (Ministries for Health, Education, Culture and Sports) was formed. The team set into motion several programs that attempt to create behavioral changes among the population. This is achieved by parallel efforts aimed at several levels:

1. Formation of awareness of the risks inherent in a harmful lifestyle and the ways to change it.
2. Creation of an environment that facilitates the maintenance of a healthy lifestyle.
3. Negative economic incentives for harmful behavior and positive incentives for healthy behavior.
4. Special attention to different ethnical subgroups.

The program's focus is on the entire population, attempting to encompass as many aspects of daily life as possible. Thus, interventions are aimed at children as well as adults, and take place in workplaces as well. Programs are enacted at all possible hierarchies starting from the national–governmental level, through municipalities, communities, families, and individuals. High-risk populations have programs tailored to their needs with the understanding and consideration of their cultural differences.

Increasing awareness

Adults
Since 2008, the health bureaus have been operating about 40 community programs every year, focused on nutrition and physical activity. Further plans are underway with the purpose of raising public awareness of proper

nutrition and increased physical activity. These include educational programs directed at educational institutions and workplaces. The Israeli "Healthy Cities Network" campaign (see below) promotes educational programs for adults regarding healthy nutrition and lifestyle.

Children

Interventional programs in children generally focus on four levels: the school, family, community, and the health care services. Consideration must be given to retention of the newly acquired skills – healthy eating habits and exercise – throughout the summer vacation.

A recent meta-analysis, which included 37 studies of child obesity prevention programs, demonstrated the effect of such interventions at reducing adiposity. However, there was a high level of heterogeneity between the programs and not all interventions were effective [17].

"Tafur Alay" (A Perfect Fit) is an Israeli health education program targeting children of a wide range of ages. It deals with three important areas of life: proper nutrition, personal hygiene, and sex education. The program, bringing together Israeli's Ministry of Education, Ministry of Health, the National Parents-Teachers Association, professional associations, and private corporations, has been running for 10 years in over 1000 schools across Israel.

The program developed educational materials and kits for grades 1–3, 3–6, and for kindergarten children. The major themes covered include the importance of breakfast, food groups, eating properly throughout the day, the importance of diversity in the foods we eat, the importance of drinking water and of regular physical activity. Special educational materials were prepared for the Arab population. These educational materials have been used by over 1000 schools and over 500 kindergartens [18].

A pilot interventional program for promoting a healthy lifestyle was operated during the school year 2009–2010 in 23 schools and kindergartens throughout the country encompassing the different cultural and ethnic groups in Israel. The purpose of the pilot was to evaluate the feasibility of such a program in Israel and its success rate. The program was directed at three levels: the school/kindergarten, the family, and the community (leisure time). A steering committee accompanied the program, defined its goals and contents, and resolved problems as they arose [19].

The goals of the program were as follow.
- *Promoting healthy nutrition:*
  - Limit intake of soft drinks. Encourage drinking water.
  - Increase intake of fruits and vegetables (five servings a day)

- ○ Recommend daily dose of low fat dairy products (at least three a day).
- ○ Eat breakfast every day.
- ○ Have family meals at least once a day with the presence of at least one parent.
- *Recommended leisure activities:*
  - ○ Limit time to watch television or play on the computer.
  - ○ Promote physical activities during leisure time.
- *Exercise:*
  - ○ At least 1 hour daily of exercise.

The principles of the program were:

- Creating a health promoting environment in the educational institutions and the community centers.
- Creating mutual commitment to the program's goals by all those involved.
- Involving the students, parents, teachers, school staff members, and the local authorities in building the program and defining its goals.
- Integrating the health promoting program into the school curriculum.
- Practical sessions, enabling the children to directly experience the recommended nutritional intake and physical activities.
- Continuous monitoring of the program while quantifying measures of failure or success.

The program was implemented in two stages: an initial stage, which included education of staff members and preparation of the educational materials, and a second stage when the program was implemented.

The interventional program lasted 6–8 months. No significant change in BMI was observed, possibly because of the short duration of the intervention. Questionnaires and interviews with school staff members revealed their significant role in the establishment of the program and in conveying the program's theme to the students. The program has been expanded to include 100 schools in the year 2011–2012.

Modifying the environment

For successful prevention it is important to create environmental conditions that promote maintaining a healthy lifestyle. This may be achieved by groups of "caring" individuals within the community as well as by governmental pressure.

The Israel Healthy City Network

The Israel Healthy City Network was founded in 1990 as part of the International Healthy Cities Network led by the World Health Organization

[20]. The primary goal of the network is to put health high on the social, economic, and political agenda of city governments. Disease prevention, health promotion, minimizing the inequality in health, and dealing with the risk factors for non-communicable diseases and injuries are additional goals.

There are currently 27 cities and four regional authorities in the network. Twenty-one additional cities are part of the network but are currently inactive. The network has promoted constructing walking lanes in all the cities in the network. All have outdoor exercise facilities and three have occasional-use courses and instruction available to the public regarding their use. Eighteen of the network participants subsidize exercise classes for children; 11 subsidize adult exercise courses. The network participants organize community-based programs for children, adolescents, and adults, about the importance of healthy nutrition and regular physical exercise. Though many of these environmental changes are implemented by motivated individuals or leaders of the community, or possibly members of the city council, it has been recognized that without legislation things are slow to improve.

Legislation
In the Knesset (Israel's legislative body) - a"health lobby," formed by many parliament members, proposed a law on November 2011 aimed at reducing the magnitude of the obesity–diabetes epidemic [21]. The law aims to encourage a healthy lifestyle in many aspects of daily life including the following.
- Enforcing the local authorities to provide or develop proper environmental infrastructure, including walking/bike routes and open exercise facilities.
- Requiring large corporations to assign one of their workers as a health coordinator. His/her role includes monitoring the nutritional quality of the food sold and served in the corporation and the exercise facilities available.
- Limitation on the sale of food having low nutritional value through vending machines and cafeterias at educational institutions.
- Limitation on the advertising of food having low nutritional value to specific media at specific hours.
- Mandatory nutritional marking of food composition at restaurants and cafeterias.

Economic incentives
Positive and negative economic incentives are a powerful means to assimilate, transmit, or convey the principles to the general public. Gradually,

as the popularity of "eating a balanced diet" increases, market forces will create strong economic incentives. Thus, some of the country's leading food chains have already begun offering low calorie dishes as part of the menu, marking the caloric content of food served, serving salad dressings on the side of the salad, and so on.

Until market forces take over, the aforementioned proposed law includes sections on creating positive and negative incentives including the following.

- Requesting the Finance Minister to consult with the Minister of Health and to form a committee evaluating possibilities of taxing companies selling unhealthy foods and creating positive economic incentives for those selling food items having high nutritional value.
- Economic incentives for "healthy" food suppliers. Incentives possibly including free advertisement offered by the local authorities or reduced taxation. The Minister of Health is required to establish criteria defining a business as a "healthy" food supplier.

Cooperation between food companies and health authorities may aid in additional initiatives. Such cooperation has already been set up in Jerusalem between one of the city's supermarket chains and Hadassah Hebrew University Hospital.

In addition, the government should create incentives for health maintenance organizations to perform individual counseling and treatment for proper nutrition and increased physical activity.

Special populations

Special programs have been established for Arab and Ethiopian populations which are categorized as high-risk populations.

Ethiopian immigrants: "Tene Briut" Program

The Jews of Ethiopia arrived in Israel in two main waves of immigration. The first in 1984–1985 and the second in 1991. The dramatic transition from Ethiopian rural living conditions to a modern urban lifestyle brought on a drastic change in the immigrants' morbidity profile. While there was a significant reduction in various types of infectious diseases there was an increase in the prevalence of chronic non-communicable diseases. BMI rose from 17–19 to 24 and, together with a decline in fitness, a sharp increase in the prevalence of type 2 diabetes was observed from 0–0.4% on arrival to Israel to 17% after 10 years in the country.

These data led to the foundation of "Tene Briut" – an interventional program for the Ethiopian immigrant population in Israel [22,23]. This program aimed to familiarize the Ethiopian population with the concepts of chronic diseases in general and diabetes in particular, preventive behavior, and preventive medicine. The program is implemented mainly by Ethiopian–Israeli medical and paraprofessionals and its activities consist of sessions that take place in a community setting.

The model was developed in several stages. The early stages focused on learning about the community from non-medical professionals (welfare, absorption workers, teachers) and from members of the community and initial gathering of information via a questionnaire based study on beliefs, perceptions, and attitudes to health and chronic diseases. Later, a steering committee was set up, composed of members of the community, government representatives, health care providers, academic and philanthropic organizations. The program was initially operated by a non-Ethiopian physician and later a group of Ethiopian immigrant nurses were trained to become Health Trustees and gradually took over the organization.

The main goals of the program were to:
- Enhance awareness and capacity of health care providers caring for the Ethiopian community;
- Provide members of the Ethiopian immigrant community with new concepts regarding health care and information about patients' rights;
- Document the health care needs of the population; and
- Influence the agenda of medical professionals and decision makers.

The program developed instructional materials suited to the immigrants' cultures and beliefs. The materials dealt with many topics including the traditional Ethiopian diet and Israeli foods – combining them to create a 'balanced diet' – physical activity, detection/diagnosing, prevention, and treatment of diabetes. Because most of the adult immigrants were illiterate, information was disseminated using educational movies combining the traditional storyteller format with music, dance, and drawing. Print media was also created. The program has ongoing assessment to ensure the issues and materials presented are relevant and understood.

The program's activities included:
- Developing a booklet for health care professionals on the issue of food and nutrition, discussing the nutritional value of traditional Ethiopian food.
- Lectures in the community setting. At the end of some sessions, blood glucose was tested – to send the message that there is no stigma attached to diabetes.
- Cookery classes.
- A monthly radio "healthy program."

- A medical telephone interpreting service has been implemented in clinics and hospitals since 2007.

Tene Briut is now a non-governmental organization working in collaboration with local and/or national organizations aiming to promote the health of the Ethiopian immigrant community in Israel.

The Arab population

The Arab population in Israel is included in the high-risk populations for the development of type 2 diabetes. In a recent survey of the northern Arab population in Israel, 70% of the surveyed people had obesity, prediabetes, or diabetes.

In the previously described interventional programs, specific educational materials for the Arab population have been created, adjusted to their cultural and social needs [24]. The Arab population are evaluated separately and the interventional programs modified on an ongoing basis.

References

1. Knowler WC, Barrett-Connor E, Fowler SE, Hamman RF, Lachin JM, Walker EA, et al; Diabetes Prevention Program Research Group. Reduction in the incidence of type 2 diabetes with lifestyle intervention or metformin. N Engl J Med 2002;346(6): 393–403.
2. Chiasson JL, Josse RG, Gomis R, Hanefeld M, Karasik A, Laakso M; STOP-NIDDM Trail Research Group. Acarbose for prevention of type 2 diabetes mellitus: the STOP-NIDDM randomised trial. Lancet 2002;359(9323):2072–7.
3. Tuomilehto J, Lindström J, Eriksson JG, Valle TT, Hämäläinen H, Ilanne-Parikka P, et al; Finnish Diabetes Prevention Study Group. Prevention of type 2 diabetes mellitus by changes in lifestyle among subjects with impaired glucose tolerance. N Engl J Med 2001;344:1343–50.
4. Saaristo T, Peltonen M, Keinänen-Kiukaanniemi S, Vanhala M, Saltevo J, Niskanen L, et al; FIN-D2D Study Group. National type 2 diabetes prevention programme in Finland: FIN-D2D. Int J Circumpolar Health 2007;66(2):101–12.
5. Saaristo T, Moilanen L, Korpi-Hyövälti E, Vanhala M, Saltevo J, Niskanen L, et al. Lifestyle intervention for prevention of type 2 diabetes in primary health care: one-year follow-up of the Finnish National Diabetes Prevention Program (FIN-D2D). Diabetes Care 2010;33(10):2146–51.
6. Paulweber B, Valensi P, Lindström J, Lalic NM, Greaves CJ, McKee M, et al. A European evidence-based guideline for the prevention of type 2 diabetes. Horm Metab Res 2010;42(Suppl 1):S3–36.
7. Herman WH. The economics of diabetes prevention. Med Clin North Am 2011; 95(2):373–84.

8. Kalter-Leibovici O, Chetrit A, Lubin F, Atamna A, Alpert G, Ziv A, et al. Adult-onset diabetes among Arabs and Jews in Israel: a population-based study. Diabet Med 2012;29(6):748–54.

9. Israel National Health Interview Survey INHIS-2, 2007–2010: Selected Findings. Israel Center for Disease Control, Ministry of Health Publication 331; 2012.

10. Manor O, Shmueli A, Ben-Yehuda A, Paltiel O, Calderon R, Jaffe DH. National Program for Quality Indicators in Community Health in Israel. Report for 2007–2009. School of Public Health and Community Medicine, Hebrew University-Hadassah. Jerusalem: Israel.

11. Pinhas-Hamiel O, Bar-Zvi E, Boyko V, Reichman B, Lerner-Geva L. Prevalence of overweight in kindergarten children in the centre of Israel: association with lifestyle habits. Child Care Health Dev 2009;35(2):147–52.

12. Mabat Youth First Israeli National Health and Nutrition Survey in 7th–12th grade students 2003–2004. The Israel Center for Disease Control Publication No. 240; December 2006.

13. Bar Dayan Y, Elishkevits K, Grotto I, Goldstein L, Goldberg A, Shvarts S, et al. The prevalence of obesity and associated morbidity among 17-year-old Israeli conscripts. Public Health 2005;119(5):385–9.

14. http://www.health.gov.il/LegislationLibrary/Bituah_01.pdf (accessed 9 March 2013).

15. Shmueli A, Bendelac J, Achdut L. Who switches sickness funds in Israel? Health Econ Policy Law 2007;2:251–65.

16. Tirosh A, Tekes-Manova D, Israeli E, Pereg D, Shochat T, Kochba I, et al. for the Israeli Diabetes Research Group. Normal fasting plasma glucose levels and type 2 diabetes in young men. N Engl J Med 2005;353:1454–62.

17. Waters E, de Silva-Sanigorski A, Hall BJ, Brown T, Campbell KJ, Gao Y, et al. Interventions for preventing obesity in children. Cochrane Database Syst Rev 2011; 12:CD001871.

18. www.tafuralay.co.il (accessed 9 March 2013).

19. The BINA program for a healthy lifestyle for children in Israel. Summary. January 2011.

20. http://www.healthycities.co.il/upload/infocenter/info_images/01082011052914 @peilut10-11.pdf (accessed 9 March 2013).

21. www.knesset.gov.il/privatelaw/data/18/3732.rtf (accessed 9 March 2013).

22. Jaffe A, Guttman N, Schuster M. The Evolution of the Tene Briut Model: Developing an Intervention Program for the Ethiopian Immigrant Population in Israel and its Challenges and Implications. Appropriate Health Care by Culturally Competent Health professionals International Workshop Report. Editor: Leon Epstein The Israel National Institute for Health Policy and Health Services Research October 2007, pp. 121–42.

23. www.tene-briut.org.il (accessed 9 March 2013).

24. Kalter-Leibovici O, Younis-Zeidan N, Atamna A, Lubin F, Alpert G, Chetrit A, et al. Lifestyle intervention in obese Arab women: a randomized controlled trial. Arch Intern Med 2010;170(11):970–6.

Index

Note:
Page numbers in *italics* refer to figures; those in **bold** refer to tables.
Abbreviations used in the index:
BMI – body mass index
FPG – fasting plasma glucose
OGTT – oral glucose tolerance test
T2D – type 2 diabetes

Prevention of Diabetes, First Edition. Edited by Peter Schwarz and Prasuna Reddy.
© 2013 John Wiley & Sons, Ltd. Published 2013 by John Wiley & Sons, Ltd.